© **Copyright 2016 by** _____
All rights reserved.

This document is geared towards providing exact and reliable information in regards to the topic and issue covered. The publication is sold with the idea that the publisher is not required to render accounting, officially permitted, or otherwise, qualified services. If advice is necessary, legal or professional, a practiced individual in the profession should be ordered.

- From a Declaration of Principles which was accepted and approved equally by a Committee of the American Bar Association and a Committee of Publishers and Associations.

In no way is it legal to reproduce, duplicate, or transmit any part of this document in either electronic means or in printed format. Recording of this publication is strictly prohibited and any storage of this document is not allowed unless with written permission from the publisher. All rights reserved.

The information provided herein is stated to be truthful and consistent, in that any liability, in terms of inattention or otherwise, by any usage or abuse of any policies, processes, or directions contained within is the solitary and utter responsibility of the recipient reader. Under no circumstances will any legal responsibility or blame be held against the publisher for any reparation, damages, or monetary loss due to the information herein, either directly or indirectly.

Respective authors own all copyrights not held by the publisher.

The information herein is offered for informational purposes solely, and is universal as so. The presentation of the information is without contract or any type of guarantee assurance.

The trademarks that are used are without any consent, and the publication of the trademark is without permission or backing by the trademark owner. All trademarks and brands within this book are for clarifying purposes only and are the owned by the owners themselves, not affiliated with any others.

Table of Contents

Introduction 6
Gluten free quick bread loaves 8
Rosemary Bread 8
Flax and sunflower seeds bread 11
Italian Parmesan Cheese Bread 14
Cheese & Herb Bread 17
Cinnamon Raisin Bread 20
Crusty Potato Bread 23
Spinach & Feta Cheese Bread 26
Cheese & Pepperoni Bread 29
Pumpkin Bread with Cream Cheese ... 32
Sweet Oatmeal Bread 35
Harvest Bread 38
Onion, Garlic, Cheese Bread 41
Dill & Cottage Cheese Bread 44
Jalapeno-Corn Bread 47
Caramelized Onion Bread 50
Vanilla Spiced Bread 53
Coconut Bread 56

Banana Nut Bread 59

Chocolate Chip Bread 62

Cranberry Walnut Bread 65

Apple Pie Bread 68

Dried berry & Almond Bread 74

Fruit Loaf 77

Maple Syrup & Spiced Bread 80

Peanut Butter & Jelly Bread 83

Gluten free bread rolls & buns 86

Pizza Crust 86

Italian Bread 88

Hot Cross Buns 91

Bread Sticks 95

Cinnamon Buns 98

Burger Buns 102

Naan Bread 105

Tomato Foccacia 108

Challah Bread 111

Sweet Dinner Rolls 114

French Baguettes 117

Onion Sandwich Rolls 120

Hawaiian Bread Rolls..........................123
Calzones..126

Introduction

The invention of bread machine has made baking incredibly easy. A bread machine not only kneads dough thoroughly, using gluten-free bread ingredients bread loaf turns out much better than prepared with traditional method. Gluten-free breads are healthier, have better texture and look, and taste better.

This cookbook catalogues two sections of gluten-free bread machine recipes. First section includes sumptuous savory and sweet quick breads and the other section contain soft and moist gluten-free bread rolls and buns. These breads are a tasty treat for the whole family.

In this cookbook, gluten-free breads are prepared using latest model of bread machine that make use of automatic knead and bake option to prepare bread. However, if your bread machine doesn't have bake option, let bread machine do mixing and kneading.

For this, select dough / knead / manual cycle to prepare dough after adding ingredients into bread machine pan. When kneading cycle ends, using moist hands transfer dough onto a clean working space, dusted with flour and punch down dough. Cover dough and let rest for 30-45 minutes or until dough doubles in size. Then shape into a loaf and place in a greased 9 by 5 inch loaf pan. Bake bread in a preheated oven at 350 degrees F for 20-25 minutes until top is nicely golden brown and inserted wooden skewer into loaf comes out clean.

Read more to explore the collection of gluten-free bread machine recipes.

Start up your bread machine and enjoy fresh gluten-free bread anytime of the day at home.

Bon Appetit!

Gluten free quick bread loaves

__Rosemary Bread__

Yield: About 1½ Pounds loaf
Bread Machine Time: 3 hours

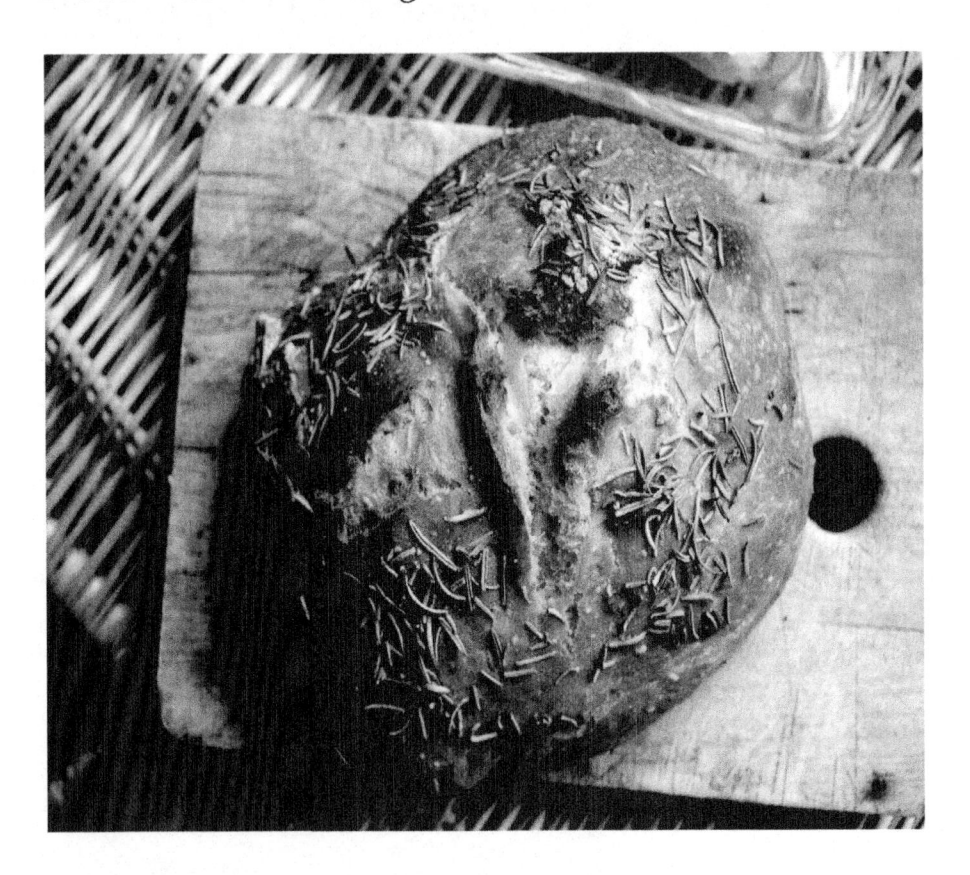

Ingredients

- 300ml (1 ¼ cups) warm water
- 60ml (¼ cup) olive oil

- 2 egg whites
- 1 tablespoon apple cider vinegar
- ½ teaspoon baking powder
- 2 teaspoons dry active yeast
- 2 tablespoons granulated sugar
- ½ teaspoon Italian seasoning
- ¼ teaspoon ground black pepper
- 1 ¼ teaspoon dried rosemary
- 200g (2 cups) gluten free almond flour / or any other gluten free flour, leveled
- 100g (1 cup) Tapioca / potato starch, leveled
- 2 teaspoons Xanthan Gum
- 1 teaspoon salt

Directions

- According to the manufacturer of your bread machine, place all the ingredients into the greased pan of bread machine.
- Select basic cycle / normal cycle / bake / quick bread / white bread setting, then select crust color either medium or light and press start to bake bread.
- In the last kneading cycle check the consistency of dough; it should be wet but thick, not like traditional bread dough. If dough is too wet, add in flour, 1 tablespoon at a time, or until dough slightly firm. If dough is too dry, add water, 1

tablespoon at a time, or until dough is slightly firm.
- When the baking cycle is finished and machine turns off, remove baked bread from pan and cool on wire rack.

Nutritional information:

150 Cal, 3g total fat, 5 mg chol., 290 mg sodium, 24g carb., 1 g fiber, 6 g protein.

Flax and sunflower seeds bread

Yield: About 1½ Pounds loaf
Bread Machine Time: 3 hours

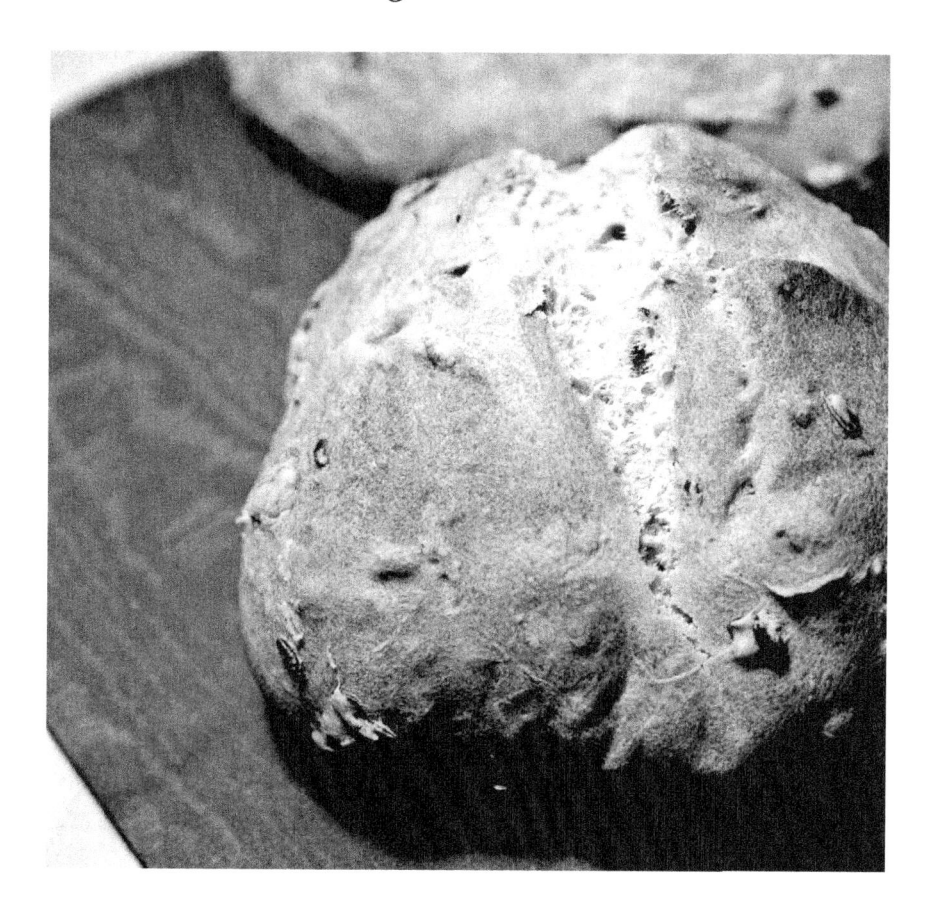

Ingredients
- 300ml (1 ¼ cups) warm water
- 60ml (¼ cup) olive oil
- 2 egg whites

- 1 tablespoon apple cider vinegar
- ½ teaspoon baking powder
- 7g (2 teaspoons) dry active yeast
- 2 tablespoons granulated sugar
- 200g (2 cups) gluten free almond flour / or any other gluten free flour, leveled
- 100g (1 cup) Tapioca / potato starch, leveled
- 2 teaspoons Xanthan Gum
- 1 teaspoon salt
- 55g (½ cup) flax seeds
- 55g (½ cup) sunflower seeds

Directions

- According to the manufacturer of your bread machine, place all the ingredients into the greased pan of bread machine except sunflower seeds.
- Select basic cycle / normal cycle / bake / quick bread / white bread setting, then select crust color either medium or light and press start.
- In the last kneading cycle check the consistency of dough; it should be wet but thick, not like traditional bread dough. If dough is too wet, add in flour, 1 tablespoon at a time, or until dough slightly firm. If dough is too dry, add water, 1 tablespoon at a time, or until dough is slightly firm.

- Add sunflower seeds 5 minutes before kneading cycle ends.
- When the baking cycle is finished and machine turns off, remove baked bread from pan and cool on wire rack.

Nutritional information:

90 Cal, 2g total fat, 5 mg chol., 180 mg sodium, 18 g carb., 2 g fiber, 4 g protein.

Italian Parmesan Cheese Bread

Yield: About 1½ Pounds loaf
Bread Machine Time: 3 hours

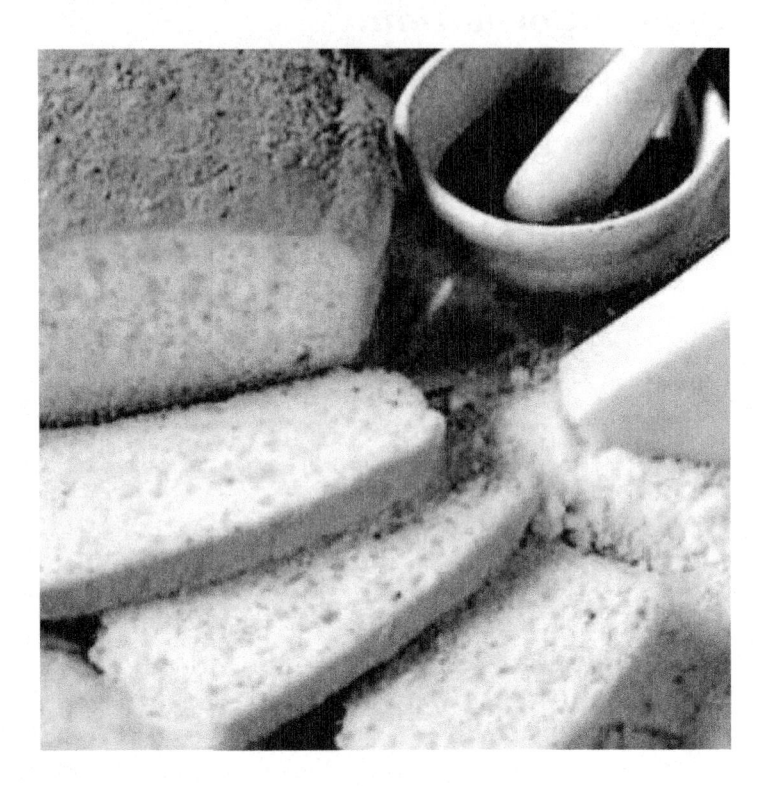

Ingredients:

- 300ml (1 ¼ cups) warm water
- 60ml (¼ cup) olive oil
- 2 egg whites
- 1 tablespoon apple cider vinegar
- ½ teaspoon baking powder

- 7g (2 teaspoons) dry active yeast
- 2 tablespoons granulated sugar
- 200g (2 cups) gluten free almond flour / or any other gluten free flour, leveled
- 100g (1 cup) Tapioca / potato starch, leveled
- 2 teaspoons Xanthan Gum
- 28g (¼ cup) grated Parmesan cheese
- 1 teaspoon salt
- 1 teaspoon Italian seasoning
- 1 teaspoon garlic powder

Directions:

- According to the manufacturer of your bread machine, place all the ingredients into the greased pan of bread machine, select basic cycle / normal cycle / bake / quick bread / white bread setting, then select crust color either medium or light and press start to bake bread.
- In the last kneading cycle check the consistency of dough; it should be wet but thick, not like traditional bread dough. If dough is too wet, add in flour, 1 tablespoon at a time, or until dough slightly firm. If dough is too dry, add water, 1 tablespoon at a time, or until dough is slightly firm.
- When the baking cycle is finished and machine turns off, remove baked bread from pan and cool on wire rack.

Nutritional information:

90 Cal, 2g total fat, 2 mg chol., 48 mg sodium, 15g carb., 1 g fiber, 2 g protein.

Cheese & Herb Bread

Yield: About 1½ Pounds loaf
Bread Machine Time: 3 hours

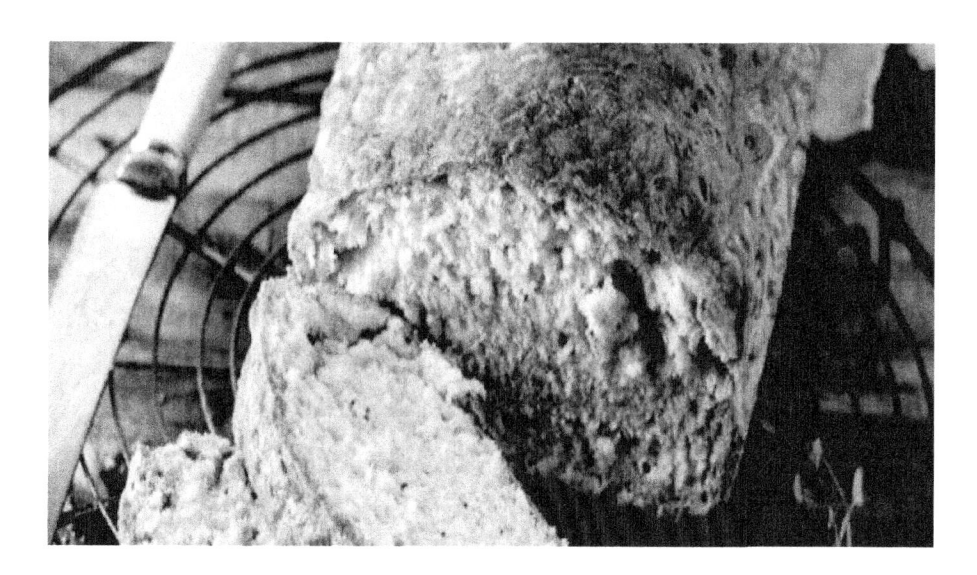

Ingredients:
- 300ml (1 ¼ cups) warm water
- 60ml (¼ cup) olive oil
- 2 egg whites
- 1 tablespoon apple cider vinegar
- ½ teaspoon baking powder
- 7g (2 teaspoons) dry active yeast
- 2 tablespoons granulated sugar
- 200g (2 cups) gluten free almond flour / or any other gluten free flour, leveled

- 100g (1 cup) Tapioca / potato starch, leveled
- 2 teaspoons Xanthan Gum
- 1 teaspoon salt
- 2 tablespoons grated Parmesan cheese
- 1 teaspoon dried marjoram
- ¾ teaspoon dried basil
- ¾ teaspoon dried oregano

Directions:

- According to the manufacturer of your bread machine, place all the ingredients into the greased pan of bread machine, select basic cycle / normal cycle / bake / quick bread / white bread setting, then select crust color either medium or light and press start to bake bread.
- In the last kneading cycle check the consistency of dough; it should be wet but thick, not like traditional bread dough. If dough is too wet, add in flour, 1 tablespoon at a time, or until dough slightly firm. If dough is too dry, add water, 1 tablespoon at a time, or until dough is slightly firm.
- When the baking cycle is finished and machine turns off, remove baked bread from pan and cool on wire rack.

Nutritional information:

150 Cal, 3g total fat, 5 mg chol., 415 mg sodium, 9g carb., 1 g fiber, 4 g protein.

Cinnamon Raisin Bread

Yield: About 1½ Pounds loaf
Bread Machine Time: 3 hours

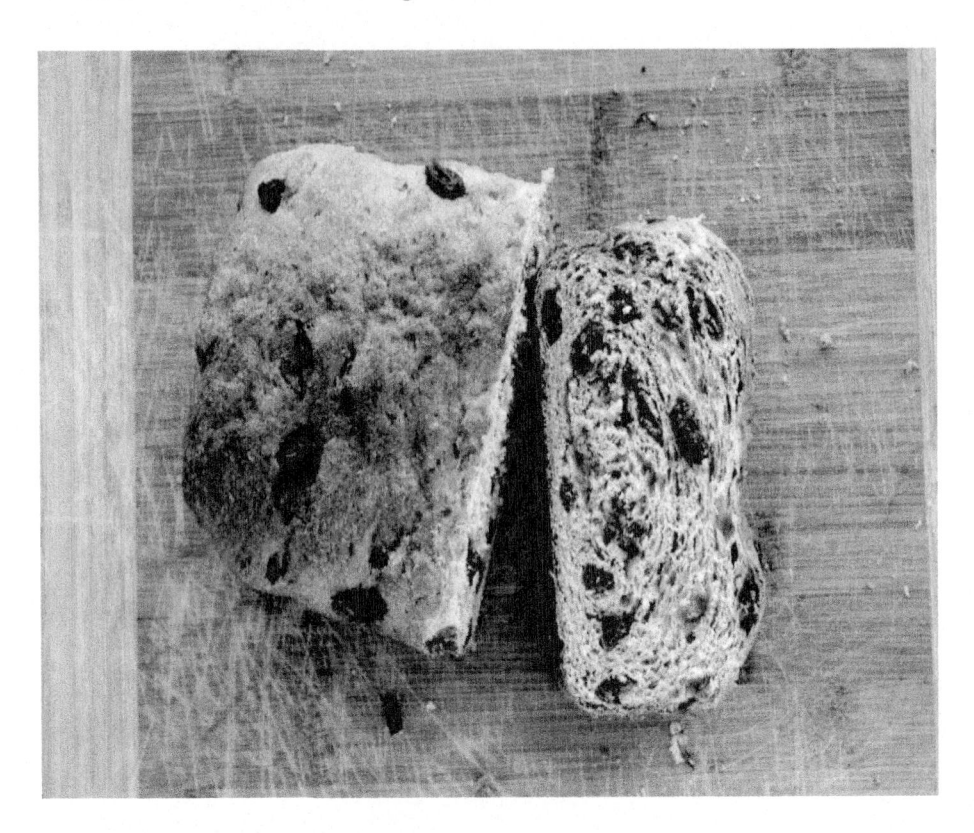

Ingredients

- 300ml (1 ¼ cups) warm water
- 60ml (¼ cup) olive oil
- 2 tablespoons honey
- 2 egg whites

- 1 tablespoon apple cider vinegar
- ½ teaspoon baking powder
- 7g (2 teaspoons) dry active yeast
- 2 tablespoons granulated sugar
- 200g (2 cups) gluten free almond flour / or any other gluten free flour, leveled
- 100g (1 cup) Tapioca / potato starch, leveled
- 2 teaspoons Xanthan Gum
- 1 teaspoon salt
- 1 teaspoon ground cinnamon
- 150g (1 cup) raisins

Directions

- According to the manufacturer of your bread machine, place all the ingredients into the greased pan of bread machine except raisins.
- Select basic cycle / normal cycle / bake / quick bread / sweet bread setting, then select crust color either medium or light and press start to bake bread.
- In the last kneading cycle check the consistency of dough; it should be wet but thick, not like traditional bread dough. If dough is too wet, add in flour, 1 tablespoon at a time, or until dough slightly firm. If dough is too dry, add water, 1 tablespoon at a time, or until dough is slightly firm.

- Add raisins 5 minutes before kneading cycle ends.
- When the baking cycle is finished and machine turns off, remove baked bread from pan and cool on wire rack.

Nutritional information

89 Cal, 1g total fat, 2 mg chol., 10 mg sodium, 13 g carb., 1 g fiber, 2.5 g protein.

Crusty Potato Bread

Yield: About 1½ Pounds loaf
Bread Machine Time: 3 hours

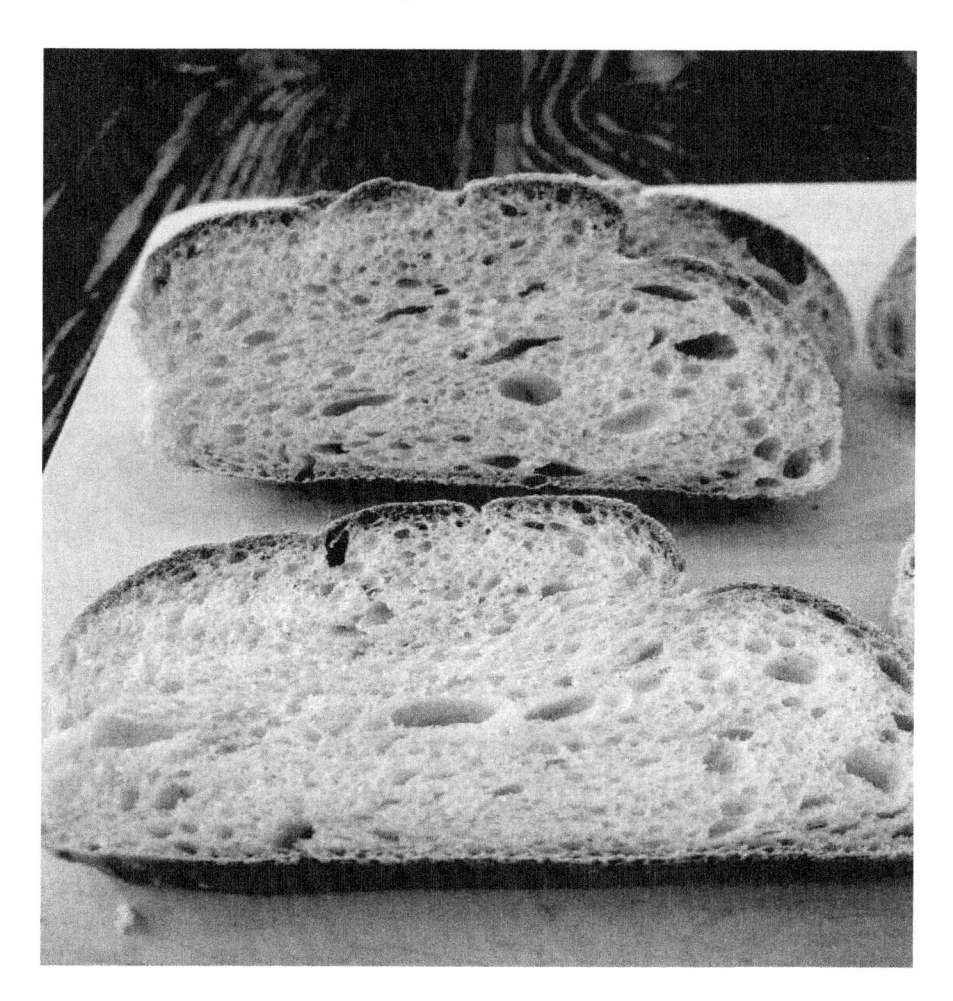

Ingredients
- 300ml (1 ¼ cups) warm water

- 60ml (¼ cup) olive oil
- 2 egg whites
- 1 tablespoon apple cider vinegar
- ½ teaspoon baking powder
- 7g (2 teaspoons) dry active yeast
- 2 tablespoons granulated sugar
- 200g (2 cups) gluten free almond flour / or any other gluten free flour, leveled
- 100g (1 cup) Tapioca / potato starch, leveled
- 2 teaspoons Xanthan Gum
- 55g (½ cup) mashed potato flakes
- 1 teaspoon salt

Directions

- According to the manufacturer of your bread machine, place all the ingredients into the greased pan of bread machine, select basic cycle / normal cycle / bake / quick bread / white bread setting, then select crust color either medium or light and press start to bake bread.
- In the last kneading cycle check the consistency of dough; it should be wet but thick, not like traditional bread dough. If dough is too wet, add in flour, 1 tablespoon at a time, or until dough slightly firm. If dough is too dry, add water, 1 tablespoon at a time, or until dough is slightly firm.

- When the baking cycle is finished and machine turns off, remove baked bread from pan and cool on wire rack.

Nutritional information:

90 Cal, 2g total fat, 5 mg chol., 232 mg sodium, 17 g carb., 1 g fiber, 3 g protein.

Spinach & Feta Cheese Bread

Yield: About 1½ Pounds loaf
Bread Machine Time: 3 hours

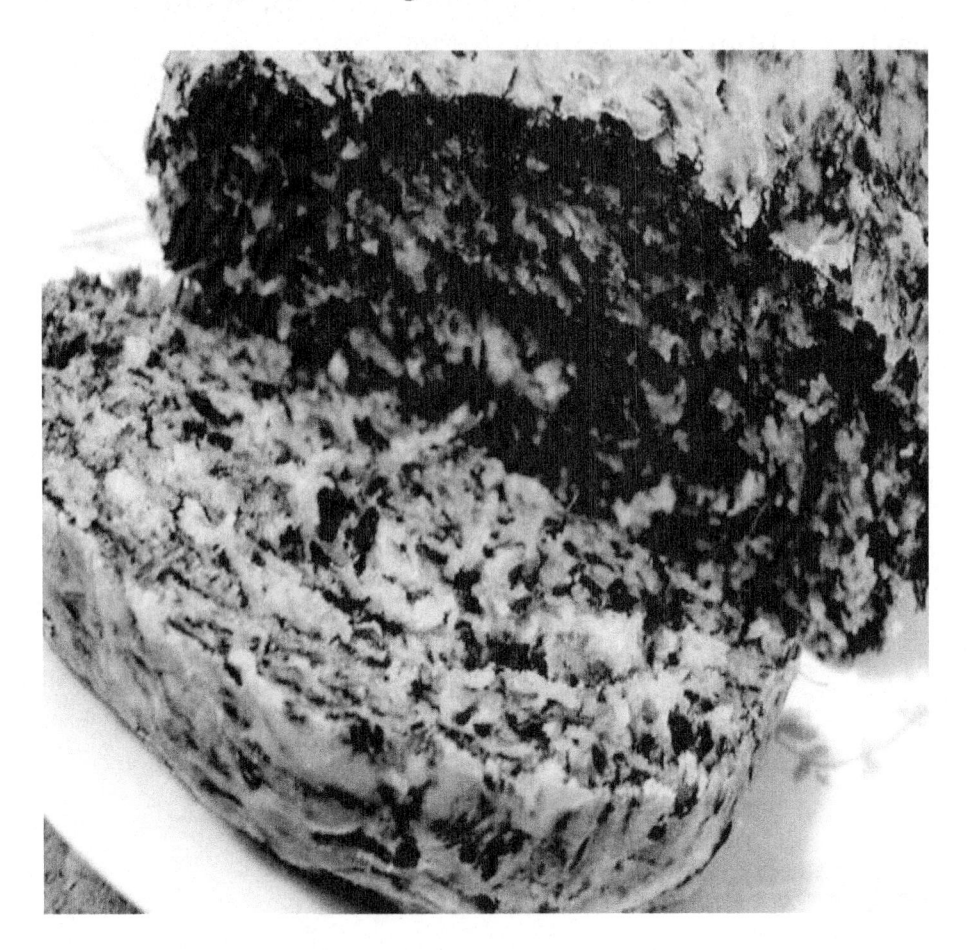

Ingredients
- 300ml (1 ¼ cups) warm water
- 60ml (¼ cup) olive oil

- 2 egg whites
- 1 tablespoon apple cider vinegar
- ½ teaspoon baking powder
- 7g (2 teaspoons) dry active yeast
- 2 tablespoons granulated sugar
- 2 teaspoons dried minced onion
- 200g (2 cups) gluten free almond flour / or any other gluten free flour, leveled
- 100g (1 cup) Tapioca / potato starch, leveled
- 2 teaspoons Xanthan Gum
- 1 teaspoon salt
- 110g (1 cup) crumbled feta cheese
- 225g (1 cup) chopped spinach

Directions

- According to the manufacturer of your bread machine, place all the ingredients into the greased pan of bread machine except cheese and spinach.
- Select basic cycle / normal cycle / bake / quick bread / white bread setting, then select crust color either medium or light and press start to bake bread.
- In the last kneading cycle check the consistency of dough; it should be wet but thick, not like traditional bread dough. If dough is too wet, add in flour, 1 tablespoon at a time, or until dough

slightly firm. If dough is too dry, add water, 1 tablespoon at a time, or until dough is slightly firm.
- Add cheese and spinach 5 minutes before kneading cycle ends.
- When the baking cycle is finished and machine turns off, remove baked bread from pan and cool on wire rack.

Nutritional information:

140 Cal, 6 g total fat, 16 mg chol., 256 mg sodium, 16 g carb., 1 g fiber, 7 g protein.

Cheese & Pepperoni Bread

Yield: About 1½ Pounds loaf
Bread Machine Time: 3 hours

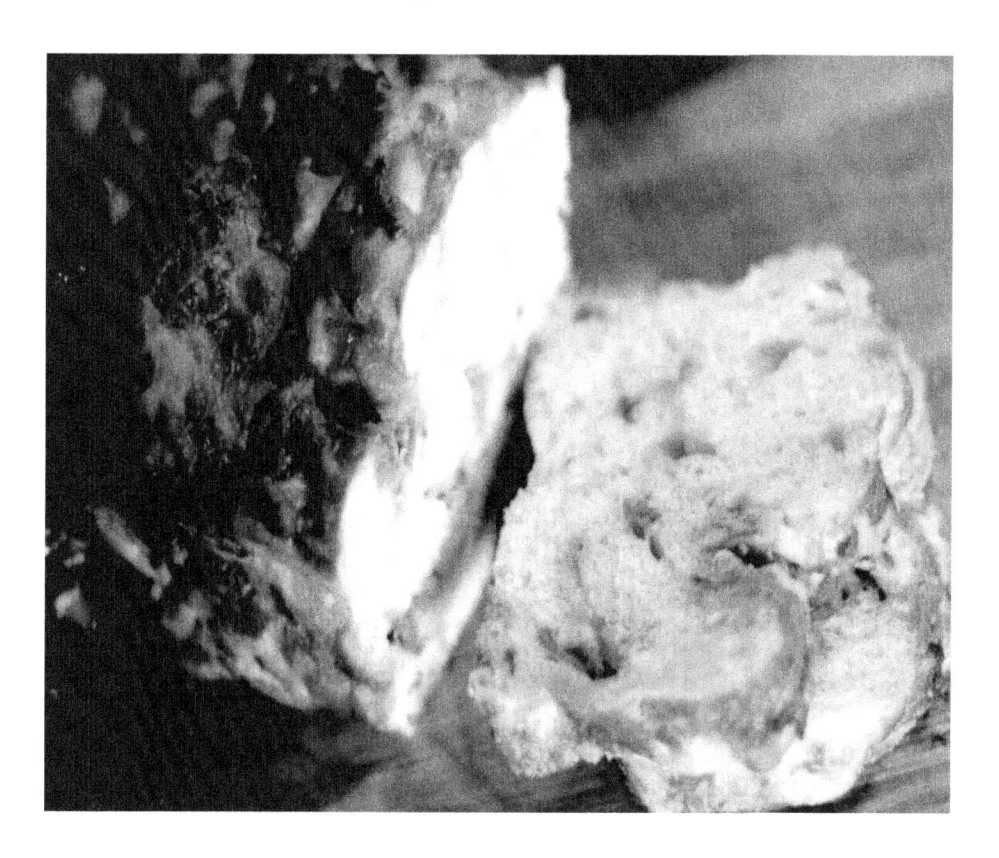

Ingredients
- 300ml (1 ¼ cups) warm water
- 60ml (¼ cup) olive oil
- 2 egg whites
- 1 tablespoon apple cider vinegar

- ½ teaspoon baking powder
- 7g (2 teaspoons) dry active yeast
- 2 tablespoons granulated sugar
- 200g (2 cups) gluten free almond flour / or any other gluten free flour, leveled
- 100g (1 cup) Tapioca / potato starch, leveled
- 2 teaspoons Xanthan Gum
- 1 teaspoon salt
- 38g (1/3 cup) shredded mozzarella cheese
- 1 teaspoon garlic powder
- 1 teaspoon dried oregano
- 55g (½ cup) diced pepperoni

Directions

- According to the manufacturer of your bread machine, place all the ingredients into the greased pan of bread machine except pepperoni.
- Select basic cycle / normal cycle / bake / quick bread / white bread setting, then select crust color either medium or light and press start to bake bread.
- In the last kneading cycle check the consistency of dough; it should be wet but thick, not like traditional bread dough. If dough is too wet, add in flour, 1 tablespoon at a time, or until dough slightly firm. If dough is too dry, add water, 1 tablespoon at a time, or until dough is slightly firm.

- Add pepperoni like nuts or other 5 minutes before kneading cycle ends.
- When the baking cycle is finished and machine turns off, remove baked bread from pan and cool on wire rack.

Nutritional information:

185 Cal, 6g total fat, 16 mg chol., 456 mg sodium, 14 g carb., 1 g fiber, 7 g protein.

Pumpkin Bread with Cream Cheese

Yield: About 1½ Pounds loaf
Bread Machine Time: 3 hours

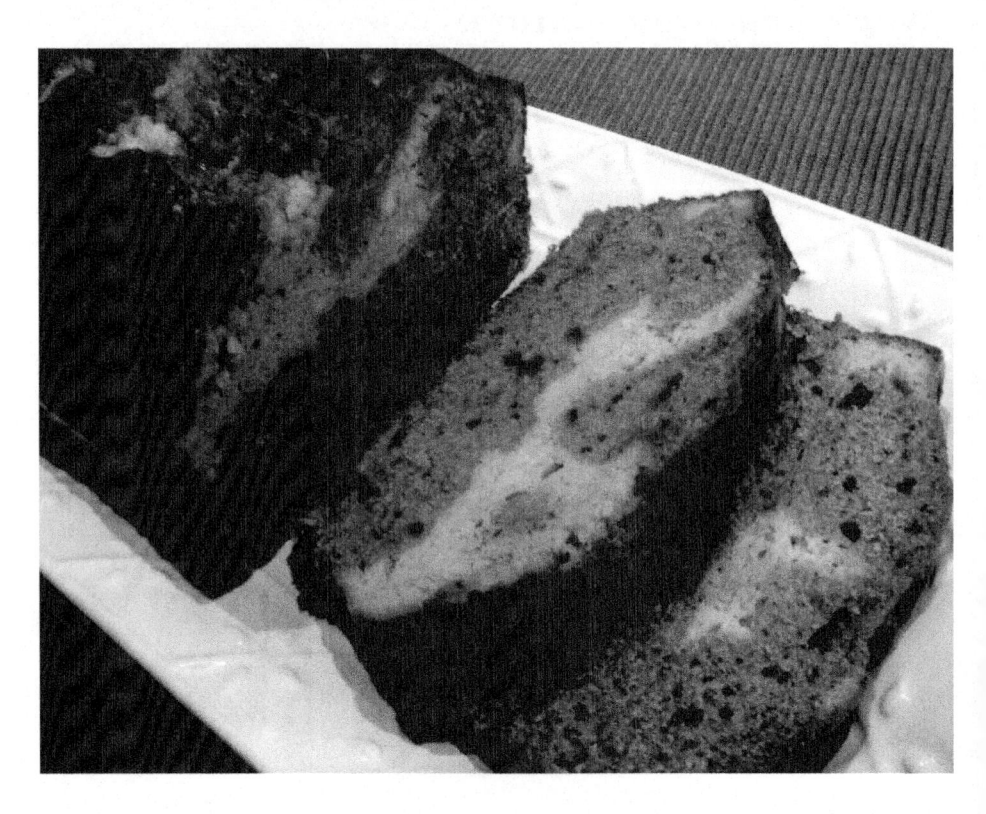

Ingredients

- 55ml (½ cup) warm water
- 60ml (¼ cup) olive oil
- 2 egg whites
- 1 tablespoon apple cider vinegar
- ½ teaspoon baking powder

- 7g (2 teaspoons) dry active yeast
- 2 tablespoons granulated sugar
- 200g (2 cups) gluten free almond flour / or any other gluten free flour, leveled
- 100g (1 cup) Tapioca / potato starch, leveled
- 2 teaspoons Xanthan Gum
- 55ml (½ cup) cream cheese, soften
- 1 teaspoon salt
- 2 teaspoons vanilla extract
- 1 cup pumpkin purée

Directions

- According to the manufacturer of your bread machine, place all the ingredients into the greased pan of bread machine, select basic cycle / normal cycle / bake / quick bread / white bread setting, then select crust color either medium or light and press start to bake bread.
- In the last kneading cycle check the consistency of dough; it should be wet but thick, not like traditional bread dough. If dough is too wet, add in flour, 1 tablespoon at a time, or until dough slightly firm. If dough is too dry, add water, 1 tablespoon at a time, or until dough is slightly firm.
- When the baking cycle is finished and machine turns off, remove baked bread from pan and cool on wire rack.

Nutritional information:

93 Cal, 13.5g total fat, 23 mg chol., 154 mg sodium, 33 g carb., 1 g fiber, 5 g protein.

Sweet Oatmeal Bread

Yield: About 1½ Pounds loaf
Bread Machine Time: 3 hours

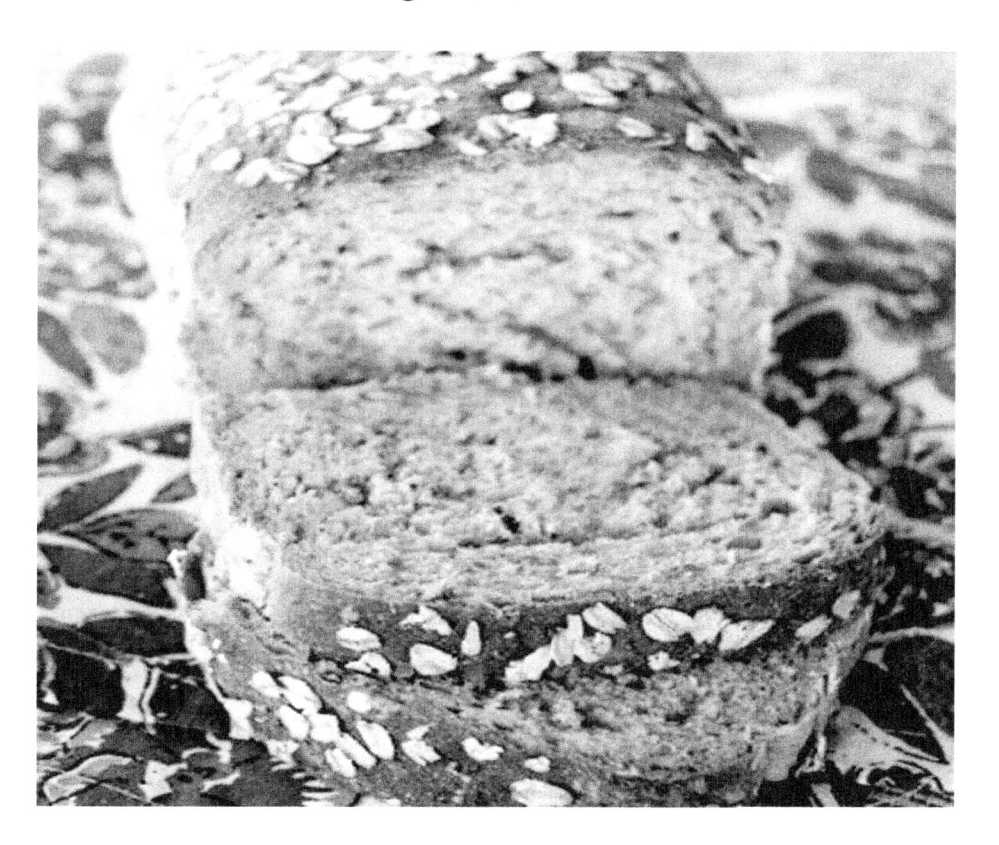

Ingredients
- 300ml (1 ¼ cups) warm water
- 60ml (¼ cup) olive oil
- 2 tablespoons honey
- 2 egg whites

- 1 tablespoon apple cider vinegar
- ½ teaspoon baking powder
- 7g (2 teaspoons) dry active yeast
- 2 tablespoons granulated sugar
- 200g (2 cups) gluten free almond flour / or any other gluten free flour, leveled
- 100g (1 cup) Tapioca / potato starch, leveled
- 2 teaspoons Xanthan Gum
- 1 teaspoon salt
- 55g (½ cup) rolled oats

Directions
- According to the manufacturer of your bread machine, place all the ingredients into the greased pan of bread machine except oats.
- Select basic cycle / normal cycle / bake / quick bread / sweet bread setting, then select crust color either medium or light and press start to bake bread.
- In the last kneading cycle check the consistency of dough; it should be wet but thick, not like traditional bread dough. If dough is too wet, add in flour, 1 tablespoon at a time, or until dough slightly firm. If dough is too dry, add water, 1 tablespoon at a time, or until dough is slightly firm.

- Add oats 5 minutes before kneading cycle ends and then kneading cycle ends, sprinkle some oats on dough.
- When the baking cycle is finished and machine turns off, remove baked bread from pan and cool on wire rack.

Nutritional information:

73 Cal, 2 g total fat, 0 mg chol., 162 mg sodium, 13.1 g carb., 1.5 g fiber, 3 g protein.

Harvest Bread

Yield: About 1½ Pounds loaf
Bread Machine Time: 3 hours

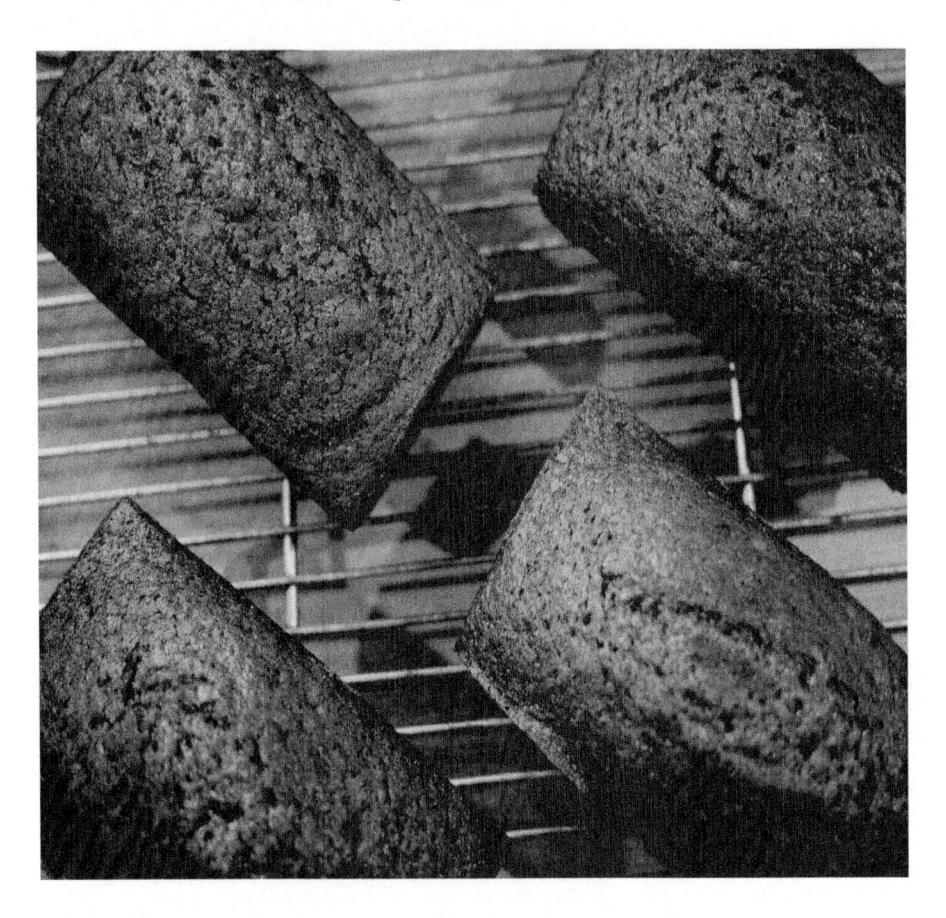

Ingredients
- 300ml (1 ¼ cups) warm water
- 60ml (¼ cup) olive oil

- 2 egg whites
- 1 tablespoon apple cider vinegar
- ½ teaspoon baking powder
- 7g (2 teaspoons) dry active yeast
- 2 tablespoons granulated sugar
- 200g (2 cups) gluten free almond flour / or any other gluten free flour, leveled
- 100g (1 cup) Tapioca / potato starch, leveled
- 2 teaspoons Xanthan Gum
- ¼ teaspoon allspice
- 1 teaspoon salt
- 55g (½ cup) pureed cooked carrots
- 55g (½ cup) pureed canned pumpkin
- 55g (½ cup) applesauce

Directions

- According to the manufacturer of your bread machine, place all the ingredients into the greased pan of bread machine, select basic cycle / normal cycle / bake / quick bread / white bread setting, then select crust color either medium or light and press start to bake bread.
- In the last kneading cycle check the consistency of dough; it should be wet but thick, not like traditional bread dough. If dough is too wet, add in flour, 1 tablespoon at a time, or until dough slightly firm. If dough is too dry, add water, 1

tablespoon at a time, or until dough is slightly firm.
- When the baking cycle is finished and machine turns off, remove baked bread from pan and cool on wire rack.

Nutritional information:

142Cal, 1 g total fat, 25 mg chol., 152 mg sodium, 32 g carb., 1 g fiber, 2.3 g protein.

Onion, Garlic, Cheese Bread

Yield: About 1½ Pounds loaf
Bread Machine Time: 3 hours

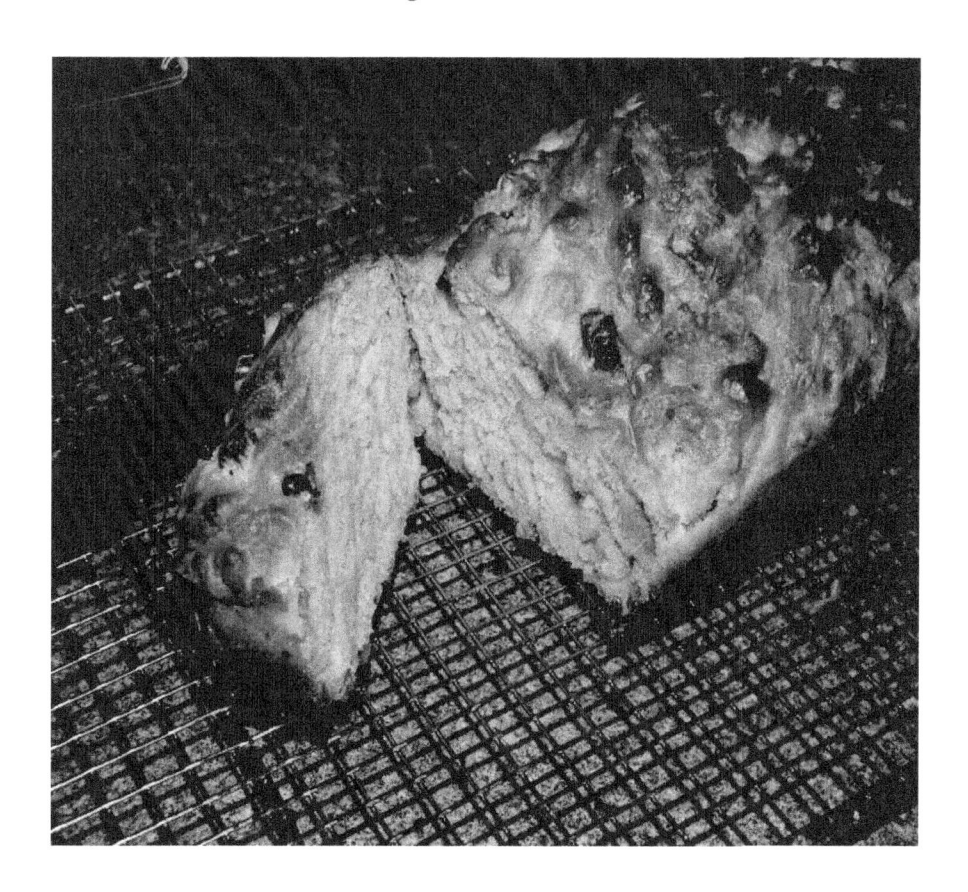

Ingredients

- 300ml (1 ¼ cups) warm water
- 60ml (¼ cup) olive oil
- 2 egg whites

- 1 tablespoon apple cider vinegar
- ½ teaspoon baking powder
- 7g (2 teaspoons) dry active yeast
- 2 tablespoons granulated sugar
- 200g (2 cups) gluten free almond flour / or any other gluten free flour, leveled
- 100g (1 cup) Tapioca / potato starch, leveled
- 2 teaspoons Xanthan Gum
- 1 teaspoon salt
- 3 tablespoons dried minced onion
- 2 teaspoons garlic powder
- 113g (1 cup) shredded mozzarella cheese

Directions

- According to the manufacturer of your bread machine, place all the ingredients into the greased pan of bread machine except minced onion, garlic powder and cheese.
- Select basic cycle / normal cycle / bake / quick bread / white bread setting, then select crust color either medium or light and press start to bake bread.
- In the last kneading cycle check the consistency of dough; it should be wet but thick, not like traditional bread dough. If dough is too wet, add in flour, 1 tablespoon at a time, or until dough slightly firm. If dough is too dry, add water, 1

tablespoon at a time, or until dough is slightly firm.
- Add minced onion, garlic powder and cheese 5 minutes before kneading cycle ends.
- When the baking cycle is finished and machine turns off, remove baked bread from pan and cool on wire rack.

Nutritional information:

160 Cal, 4 g total fat, 10mg chol., 280 mg sodium, 25 g carb., 1 g fiber, 6 g protein.

Dill & Cottage Cheese Bread

Yield: About 1½ Pounds loaf
Bread Machine Time: 3 hours

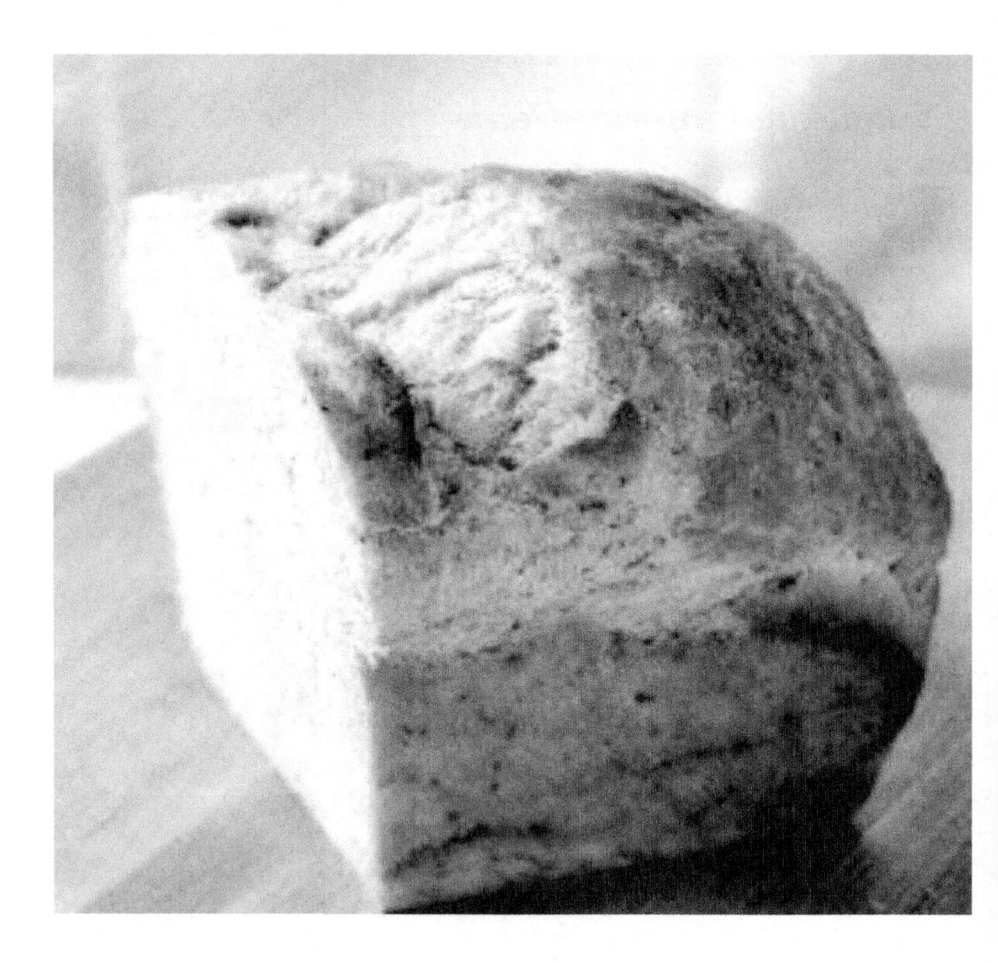

Ingredients
- 300ml (1 ¼ cups) warm water
- 60ml (¼ cup) olive oil

- 2 egg whites
- 1 tablespoon apple cider vinegar
- ½ teaspoon baking powder
- 7g (2 teaspoons) dry active yeast
- 2 tablespoons granulated sugar
- 200g (2 cups) gluten free almond flour / or any other gluten free flour, leveled
- 100g (1 cup) Tapioca / potato starch, leveled
- 2 teaspoons Xanthan Gum
- 1 teaspoon salt
- 1 teaspoon dried minced onion
- 1 tablespoon dill seed
- 75g (2/3 cup) cottage cheese

Directions

- According to the manufacturer of your bread machine, place all the ingredients into the greased pan of bread machine, select basic cycle / normal cycle / bake / quick bread / white bread setting, then select crust color either medium or light and press start to bake bread.
- In the last kneading cycle check the consistency of dough; it should be wet but thick, not like traditional bread dough. If dough is too wet, add in flour, 1 tablespoon at a time, or until dough slightly firm. If dough is too dry, add water, 1 tablespoon at a time, or until dough is slightly firm.

- When the baking cycle is finished and machine turns off, remove baked bread from pan and cool on wire rack.

Nutritional information:

137 Cal, 1.2 g total fat, 20 mg chol., 356 mg sodium, 24 g carb., 1 g fiber, 6.6 g protein.

Jalapeno-Corn Bread

Yield: About 1½ Pounds loaf
Bread Machine Time: 3 hours

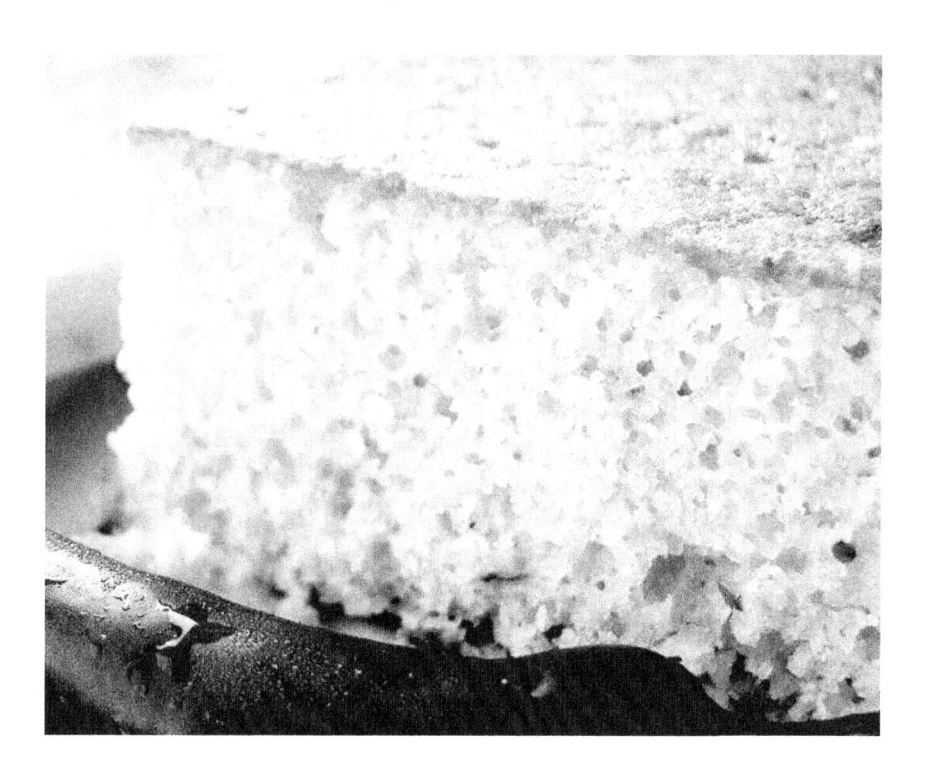

Ingredients
- 300ml (1 ¼ cups) warm water
- 60ml (¼ cup) olive oil
- 2 egg whites
- 1 tablespoon apple cider vinegar
- ½ teaspoon baking powder
- 7g (2 teaspoons) dry active yeast

- 2 tablespoons granulated sugar
- 200g (2 cups) gluten free almond flour / or any other gluten free flour, leveled
- 75g (2/3 cup) Tapioca / potato starch, leveled
- 38g (1/3 cup) cornmeal
- 2 teaspoons Xanthan Gum
- 1 teaspoon salt
- 75g (2/3 cup) frozen corn, thawed
- 1 tablespoon chopped jalapeno pepper

Directions

- According to the manufacturer of your bread machine, place all the ingredients into the greased pan of bread machine, select basic cycle / normal cycle / bake / quick bread / white bread setting, then select crust color either medium or light and press start to bake bread.
- In the last kneading cycle check the consistency of dough; it should be wet but thick, not like traditional bread dough. If dough is too wet, add in flour, 1 tablespoon at a time, or until dough slightly firm. If dough is too dry, add water, 1 tablespoon at a time, or until dough is slightly firm.
- When the baking cycle is finished and machine turns off, remove baked bread from pan and cool on wire rack.

Nutritional information:

163 Cal, 8g total fat, 32 mg chol., 250 mg sodium, 21 g carb., 2.1 g fiber, 4.2 g protein.

Caramelized Onion Bread

Yield: About 1½ Pounds loaf
Bread Machine Time: 3 hours

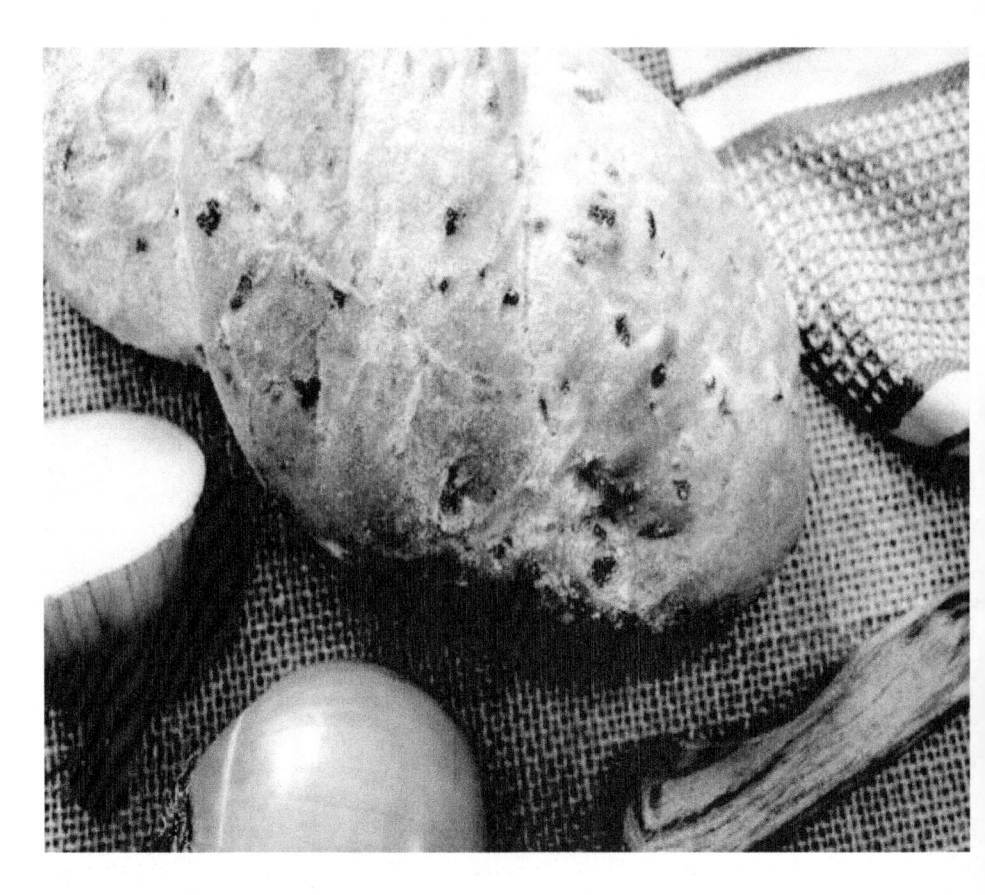

Ingredients

- 300ml (1 ¼ cups) warm water
- 60ml (¼ cup) olive oil
- 2 egg whites

- 1 tablespoon apple cider vinegar
- ½ teaspoon baking powder
- 1 medium onion
- 1 tablespoon fat-free butter
- 7g (2 teaspoons) dry active yeast
- 2 tablespoons granulated sugar
- 200g (2 cups) gluten free almond flour / or any other gluten free flour, leveled
- 100g (1 cup) Tapioca / potato starch, leveled
- 2 teaspoons Xanthan Gum
- 1 teaspoon salt

Directions

- Peel onion and slice thinly. Place a non-stick skillet pan over medium-low flame, add 1 tablespoon butter and heat until melt. Add onions and cook for 10-15 minutes or until onions are nicely brown and caramelized, stir occasionally.
- According to the manufacturer of your bread machine, place all the ingredients in to the greased pan of bread machine except caramelized onion.
- Select basic cycle / normal cycle / bake / quick bread / white bread setting, then select crust color either medium or light and press start to bake bread.

- In the last kneading cycle check the consistency of dough; it should be wet but thick, not like traditional bread dough. If dough is too wet, add in flour, 1 tablespoon at a time, or until dough slightly firm. If dough is too dry, add water, 1 tablespoon at a time, or until dough is slightly firm.
- Add caramelized onion 5 minutes before kneading cycle ends.
- When the baking cycle is finished and machine turns off, remove baked bread from pan and cool on wire rack.

Nutritional information:

106 Cal, 1.5 g total fat, 15 mg chol., 150 mg sodium, 20.3 g carb., 1.7 g fiber, 3.3 g protein.

Vanilla Spiced Bread

Yield: About 1½ Pounds loaf
Bread Machine Time: 3 hours

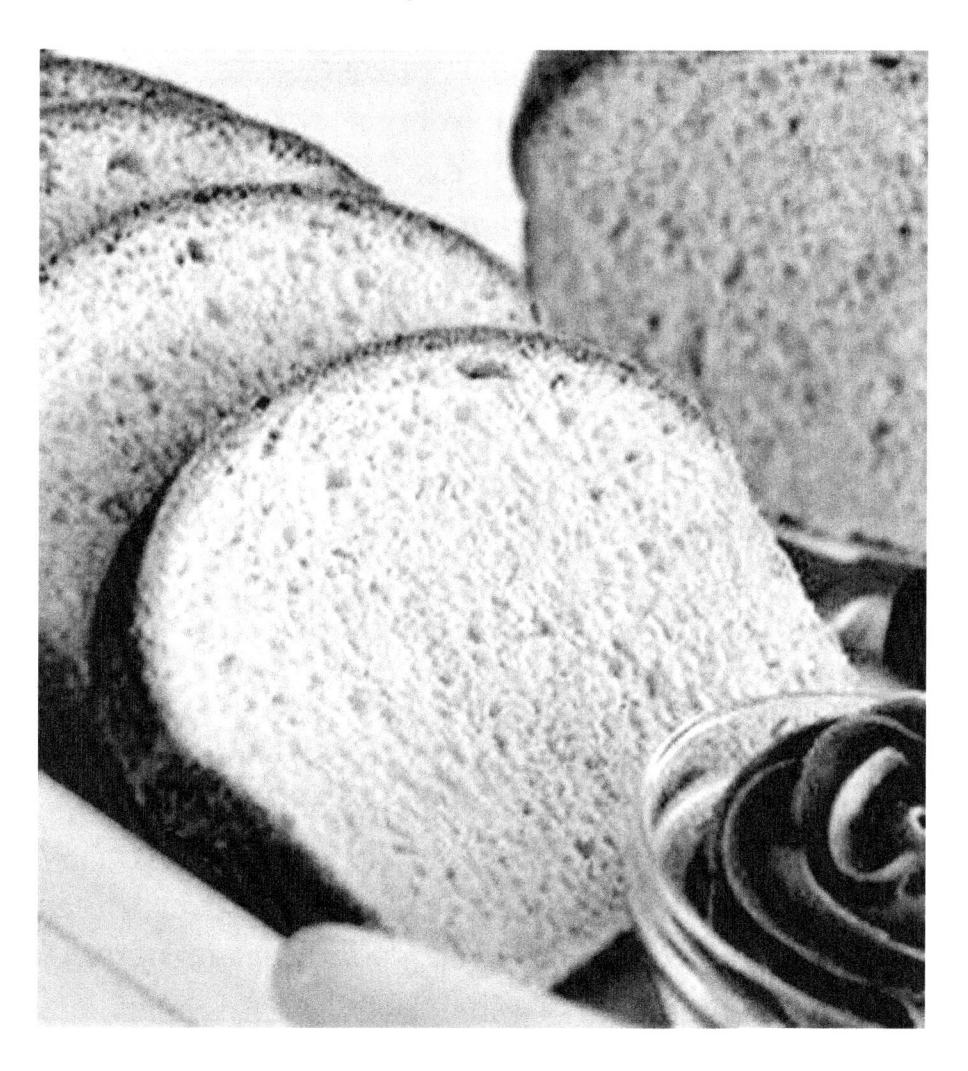

Ingredients
- 300ml (1 ¼ cups) milk, unsweetened
- 60ml (¼ cup) olive oil
- 1 tablespoon vanilla, unsweetened
- 2 egg whites
- 1 tablespoon apple cider vinegar
- ½ teaspoon baking powder
- 7g (2 teaspoons) dry active yeast
- 2 tablespoons granulated sugar
- 55g (¼ cup) brown sugar, packed
- 200g (2 cups) gluten free almond flour / or any other gluten free flour, leveled
- 100g (1 cup) Tapioca / potato starch, leveled
- 2 teaspoons Xanthan Gum
- 1 teaspoon salt
- ¼ teaspoon ground coriander

Directions
- According to the manufacturer of your bread machine, place all the ingredients into the greased pan of bread machine, select basic cycle / normal cycle / bake / quick bread / sweet bread setting, then select crust color either medium or light and press start to bake bread.
- In the last kneading cycle check the consistency of dough; it should be wet but thick, not like

traditional bread dough. If dough is too wet, add in flour, 1 tablespoon at a time, or until dough slightly firm. If dough is too dry, add water, 1 tablespoon at a time, or until dough is slightly firm.
- When the baking cycle is finished and machine turns off, remove baked bread from pan and cool on wire rack.

Nutritional information:

186 Cal, 8 g total fat, 0 mg chol., 150 mg sodium, 24 g carb., 1 g fiber, 4 g protein.

Coconut Bread

Yield: About 1½ Pounds loaf
Bread Machine Time: 3 hours

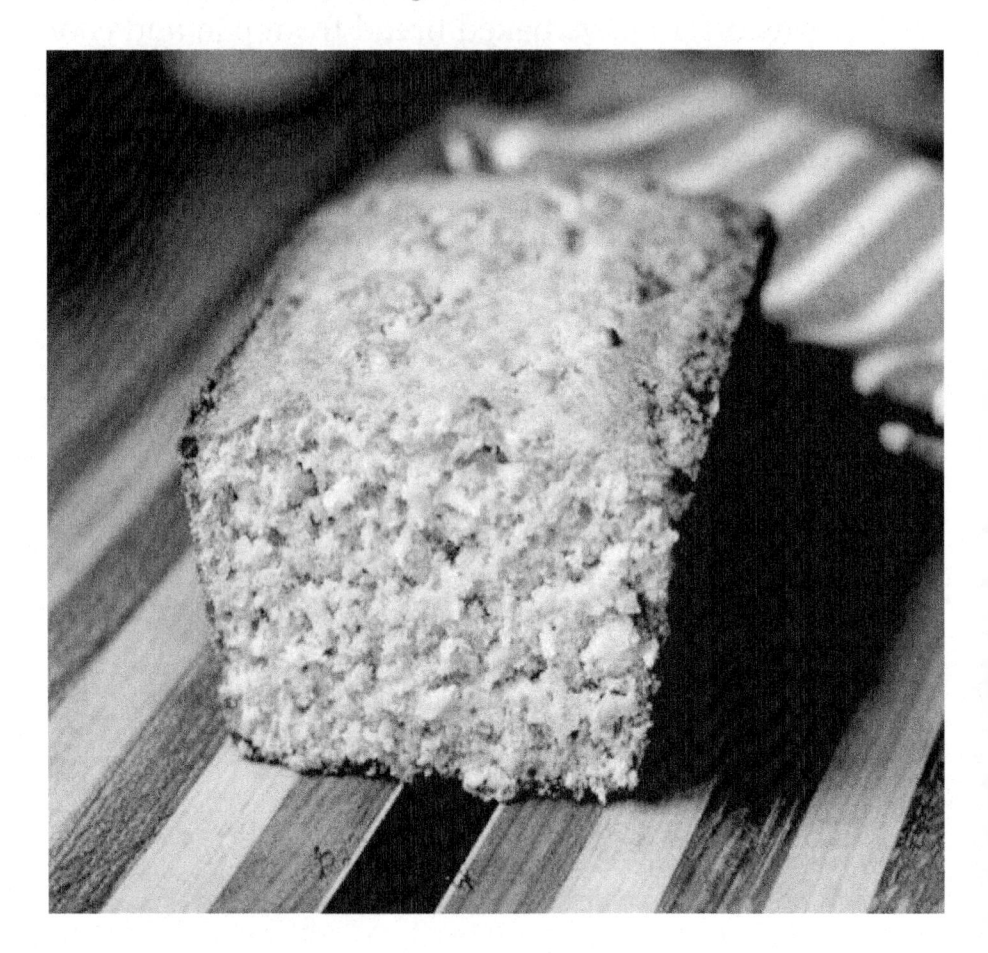

Ingredients

- 300ml (1 ¼ cups) coconut milk, unsweetened
- 60ml (¼ cup) olive oil

- 1 ½ teaspoons coconut extract
- 2 egg whites
- 1 tablespoon apple cider vinegar
- ½ teaspoon baking powder
- 7g (2 teaspoons) dry active yeast
- 2 tablespoons granulated sugar
- 37g (1/3 cup) shredded coconut
- 200g (2 cups) gluten free almond flour / or any other gluten free flour, leveled
- 100g (1 cup) Tapioca / potato starch, leveled
- 2 teaspoons Xanthan Gum
- 1 teaspoon salt

Directions
- According to the manufacturer of your bread machine, place all the ingredients into the greased pan of bread machine.
- Select basic cycle / normal cycle / bake / quick bread / sweet bread setting, then select crust color either medium or light and press start to bake bread.
- In the last kneading cycle check the consistency of dough; it should be wet but thick, not like traditional bread dough. If dough is too wet, add in flour, 1 tablespoon at a time, or until dough slightly firm. If dough is too dry, add water, 1 tablespoon at a time, or until dough is slightly firm.

- When the baking cycle is finished and machine turns off, remove baked bread from pan and cool on wire rack.

Nutritional information:

178 Cal, 3g total fat,18 mg chol., 228 mg sodium, 35 g carb., 1 g fiber, 4 g protein.

Banana Nut Bread

Yield: About 1½ Pounds loaf
Bread Machine Time: 3 hours

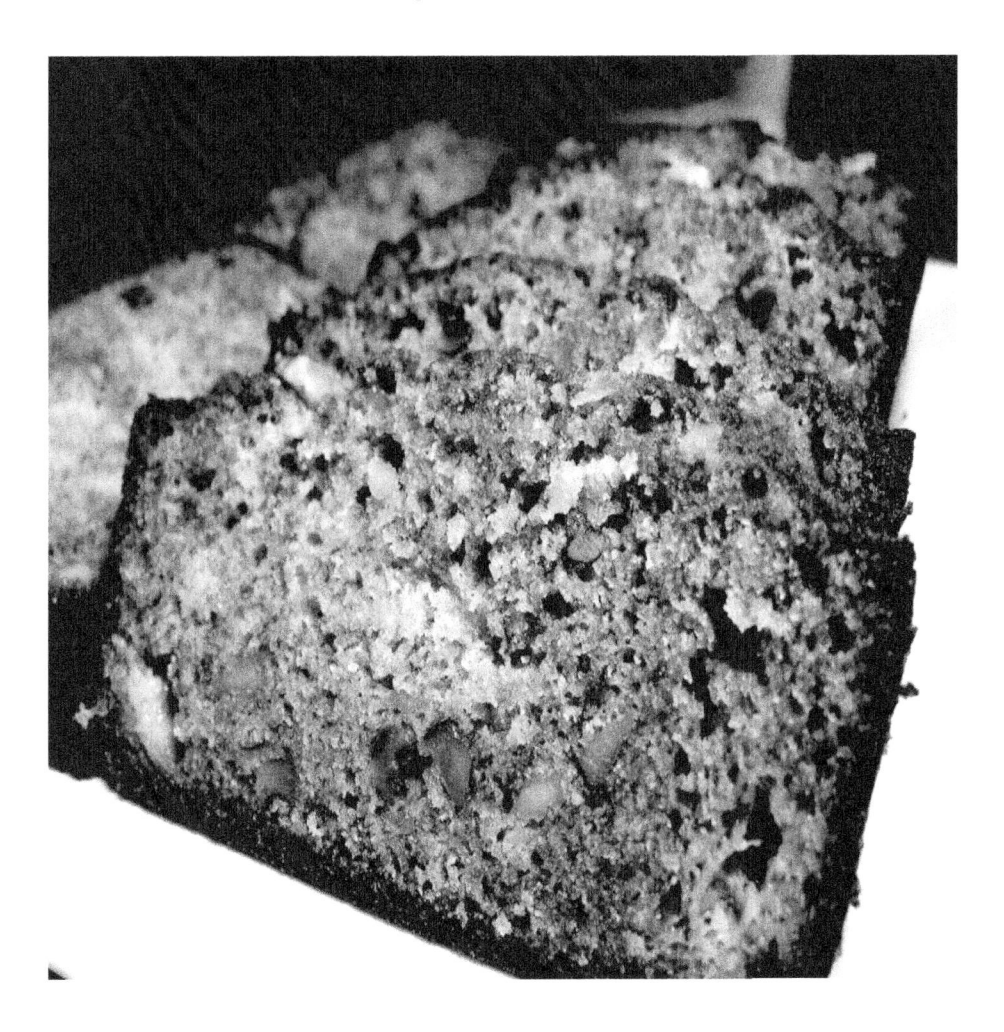

Ingredients
- 300ml (1 ¼ cups) milk, unsweetened
- 56g (½ cup) honey
- 60ml (¼ cup) olive oil
- 2 egg whites
- 75g (2/3 cup) mashed bananas
- 1 tablespoon apple cider vinegar
- ½ teaspoon baking powder
- 7g (2 teaspoons) dry active yeast
- 2 tablespoons granulated sugar
- 200g (2 cups) gluten free almond flour / or any other gluten free flour, leveled
- 100g (1 cup) Tapioca / potato starch, leveled
- 2 teaspoons Xanthan Gum
- 1 teaspoon salt
- 56g (½ cup) chopped walnuts

Directions
- According to the manufacturer of your bread machine, place all the ingredients into the greased pan of bread machine.
- Select basic cycle / normal cycle / bake / quick bread / sweet bread setting, then select crust color either medium or light and press start to bake bread.

- In the last kneading cycle check the consistency of dough; it should be wet but thick, not like traditional bread dough. If dough is too wet, add in flour, 1 tablespoon at a time, or until dough slightly firm. If dough is too dry, add water, 1 tablespoon at a time, or until dough is slightly firm.
- When the baking cycle is finished and machine turns off, remove baked bread from pan and cool on wire rack.

Nutritional information:

141 Cal, 7 g total fat, 7 mg chol., 275 mg sodium, 30 g carb., 1 g fiber, 3 g protein.

Chocolate Chip Bread

Yield: About 1½ Pounds loaf
Bread Machine Time: 3 hours

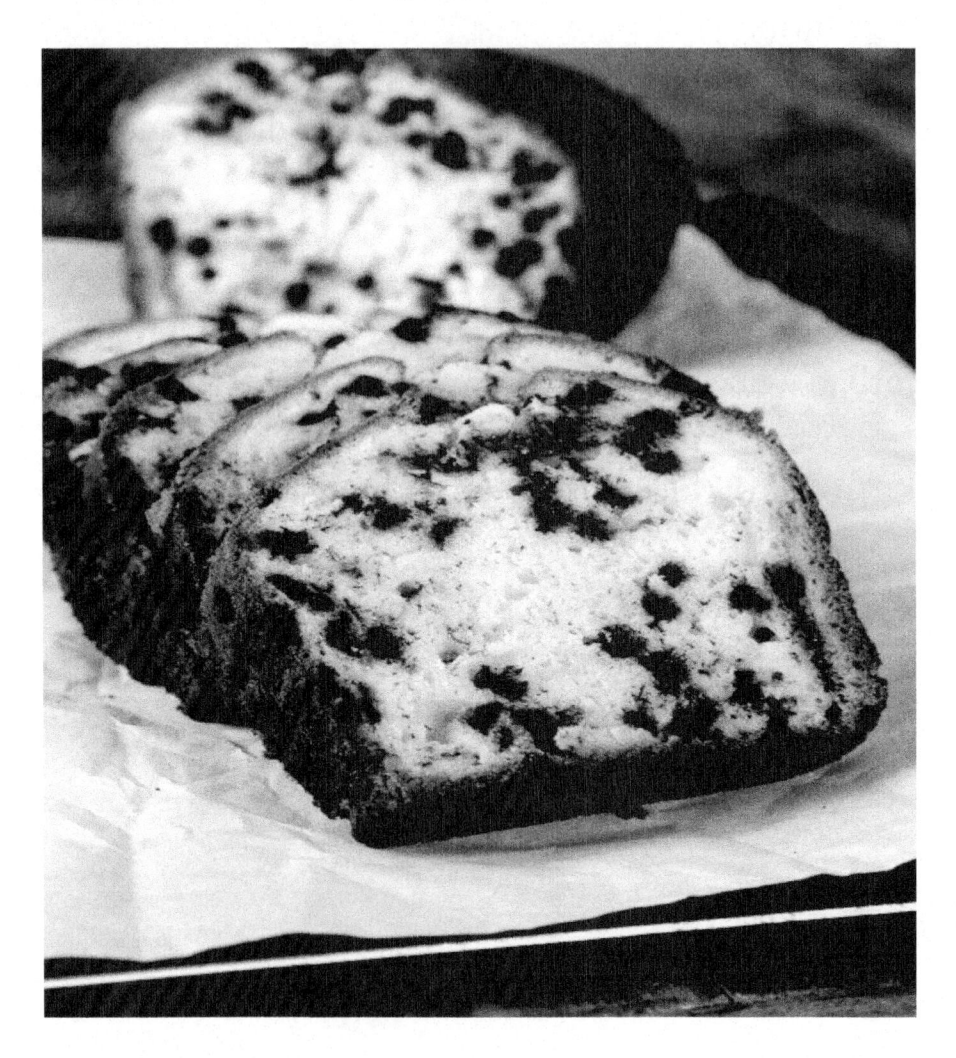

Ingredients
- 300ml (1 ¼ cups) warm water
- 60ml (¼ cup) olive oil
- 2 egg whites
- 1 tablespoon apple cider vinegar
- ½ teaspoon baking powder
- 7g (2 teaspoons) dry active yeast
- 2 tablespoons granulated sugar
- 200g (2 cups) gluten free almond flour / or any other gluten free flour, leveled
- 100g (1 cup) Tapioca / potato starch, leveled
- 2 teaspoons Xanthan Gum
- 1 teaspoon salt

Directions
- According to the manufacturer of your bread machine, into the greased pan of bread machine place all the ingredients except chocolate chips.
- Select basic cycle / normal cycle / bake / quick bread / sweet bread setting, then select crust color either medium or light and press start to bake bread.
- In the last kneading cycle check the consistency of dough; it should be wet but thick, not like traditional bread dough. If dough is too wet, add in flour, 1 tablespoon at a time, or until dough

slightly firm. If dough is too dry, add water, 1 tablespoon at a time, or until dough is slightly firm.
- Add walnuts 5 minutes before kneading cycle ends.
- When the baking cycle is finished and machine turns off, remove baked bread from pan and cool on wire rack.
- Remove baked bread from pan and cool on wire rack.

Nutritional information:

186 Cal, 9 g total fat, 15 mg chol., 150 mg sodium, 19 g carb., 1 g fiber, 4 g protein.

Cranberry Walnut Bread

Yield: About 1½ Pounds loaf
Bread Machine Time: 3 hours

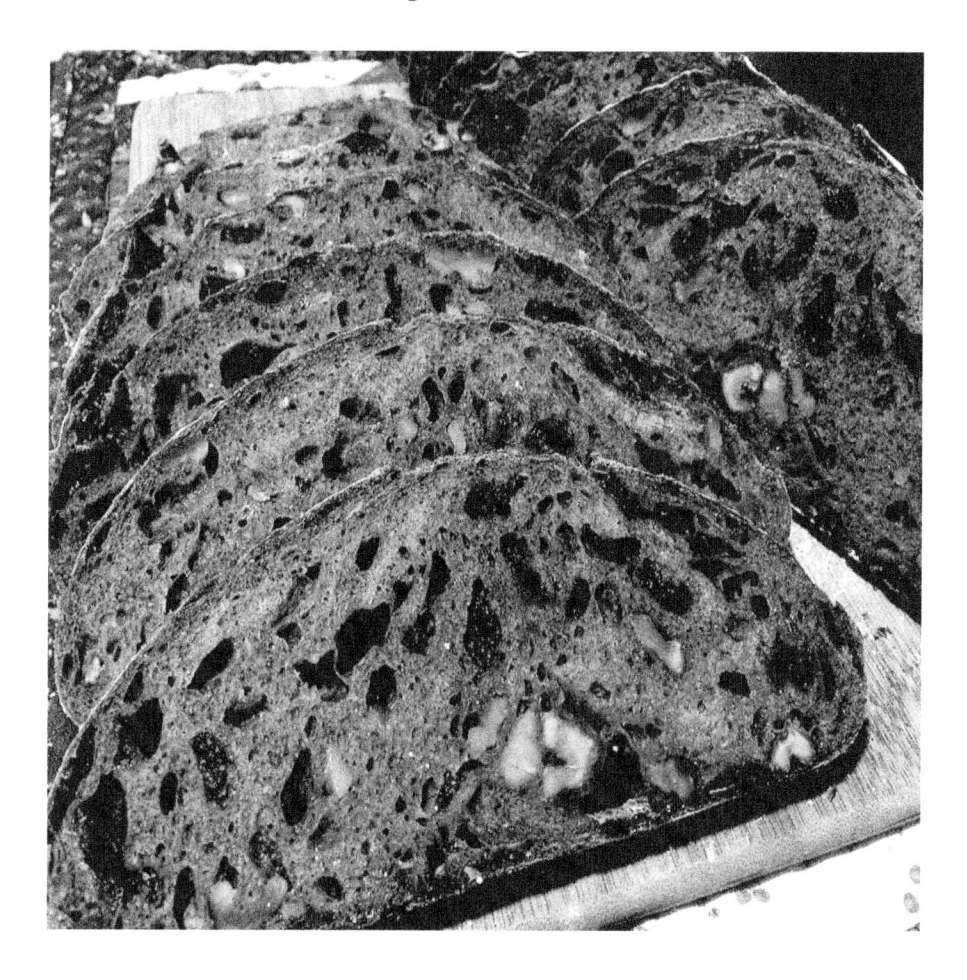

Ingredients
- 300ml (1 ¼ cups) buttermilk
- 3 tablespoons honey

- 3 tablespoons margarine
- 2 egg whites
- 1 tablespoon apple cider vinegar
- ½ teaspoon baking powder
- 7g (2 teaspoons) dry active yeast
- 200g (2 cups) gluten free almond flour / or any other gluten free flour, leveled
- 100g (1 cup) Tapioca /potato starch, leveled
- 2 teaspoons Xanthan Gum
- ½ teaspoon ground cinnamon
- 22.5g (¼ cup) rolled oats
- 90g (¾ cup) dried cranberries
- 60g (½ cup) chopped walnuts

Directions

- According to the manufacturer of your bread machine, into the greased pan of bread machine place all the ingredients except cranberries and walnuts.
- Select basic cycle / normal cycle / bake / quick bread / sweet bread setting, then select crust color either medium or light and press start to bake bread.
- In the last kneading cycle check the consistency of dough; it should be wet but thick, not like traditional bread dough. If dough is too wet, add in flour, 1 tablespoon at a time, or until dough slightly firm. If dough is too dry, add water, 1

tablespoon at a time, or until dough is slightly firm.
- Add cranberries and walnuts 5 minutes before kneading cycle ends.
- When the baking cycle is finished and machine turns off, remove baked bread from pan and cool on wire rack.
- Remove baked bread from pan and cool on wire rack.

Nutritional information:

120 Cal, 4g total fat, 13 mg chol., 140 mg sodium, 19 g carb., 1 g fiber, 2 g protein.

Apple Pie Bread

Yield: About 1½ Pounds loaf
Bread Machine Time: 3 hours

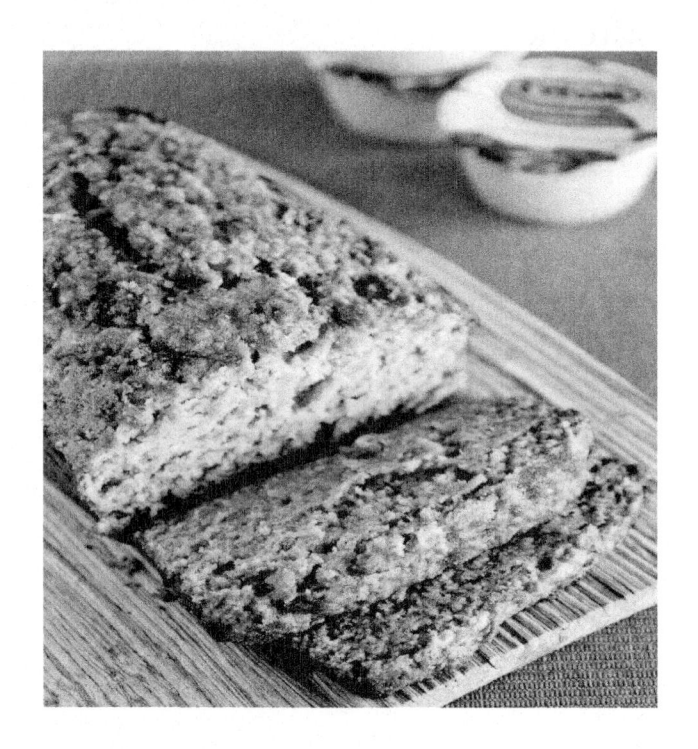

Ingredients
- 300ml (1 ¼ cups) buttermilk
- 60ml (¼ cup) olive oil
- 3 tablespoons honey
- 2 egg whites
- 1 tablespoon apple cider vinegar

- ½ teaspoon baking powder 7g (2 teaspoons) dry active yeast
- 200g (2 cups) gluten free almond flour / or any other gluten free flour, leveled
- 100g (1 cup) Tapioca / potato starch, leveled
- 2 teaspoons Xanthan Gum
- 275g (1 ¼ cups) apple pie filling

Directions

- According to the manufacturer of your bread machine, into the greased pan of bread machine place all the ingredients.
- Select basic cycle / normal cycle / bake / quick bread / sweet bread setting, then select crust color either medium or light and press start to bake bread.
- In the last kneading cycle check the consistency of dough; it should be wet but thick, not like traditional bread dough. If dough is too wet, add in flour, 1 tablespoon at a time, or until dough slightly firm. If dough is too dry, add water, 1 tablespoon at a time, or until dough is slightly firm.
- When the baking cycle is finished and machine turns off, remove baked bread from pan and cool on wire rack.

Nutritional information:

100 Cal, 18 g total fat, 5 mg chol., 100 mg sodium, 20 g carb., 1 g fiber, 2 g protein.

Sweet Orange Bread

Yield: About 1½ Pounds loaf
Bread Machine Time: 3 hours

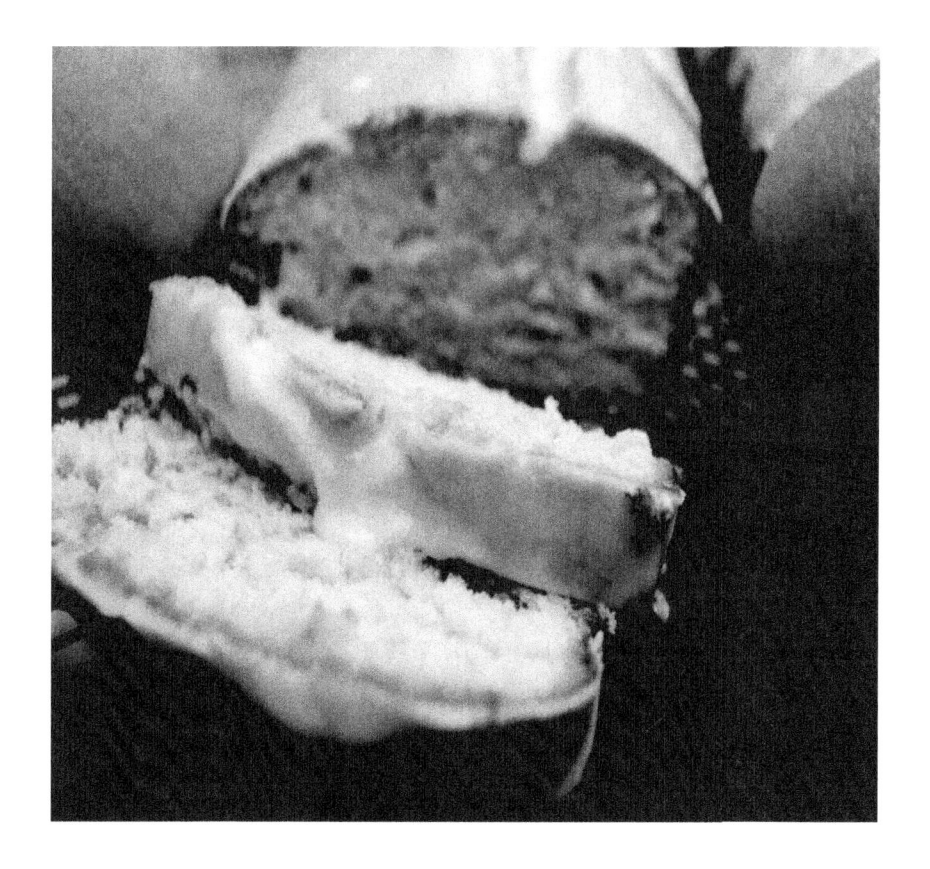

Ingredients
- 300ml (1 ¼ cups) warm water
- 60ml (¼ cup) olive oil

- 3 tablespoons honey
- 2 egg whites
- 3 tablespoons orange juice concentrate
- 1 tablespoon apple cider vinegar
- ½ teaspoon baking powder
- 7g (2 teaspoons) dry active yeast
- 200g (2 cups) gluten free almond flour / or any other gluten free flour, leveled
- 100g (1 cup) Tapioca / potato starch, leveled
- 2 teaspoons Xanthan Gum
- 1 teaspoon salt
- ½ teaspoon orange peel

For the glaze:

- 94g (¾ cup) powdered sugar
- 2 tablespoons orange juice

Directions

- According to the manufacturer of your bread machine, into the greased pan of bread machine place all the ingredients.
- Select basic cycle / normal cycle / bake / quick bread / sweet bread setting, then select crust color either medium or light and press start to bake bread.
- In the last kneading cycle check the consistency of dough; it should be wet but thick, not like

traditional bread dough. If dough is too wet, add in flour, 1 tablespoon at a time, or until dough slightly firm. If dough is too dry, add water, 1 tablespoon at a time, or until dough is slightly firm.
- In the meantime, prepare glaze. Stir together orange juice and sugar until combine.
- When the baking cycle is finished and machine turns off, remove baked bread from pan and cool on wire rack.
- Spoon prepared orange glaze over loaf and slice to serve.

Nutritional information:

175 Cal, 3g total fat, 30 mg chol., 270 mg sodium, 33g carb., 1 g fiber, 5 g protein.

Dried berry & Almond Bread

Yield: About 1½ Pounds loaf
Bread Machine Time: 3 hours

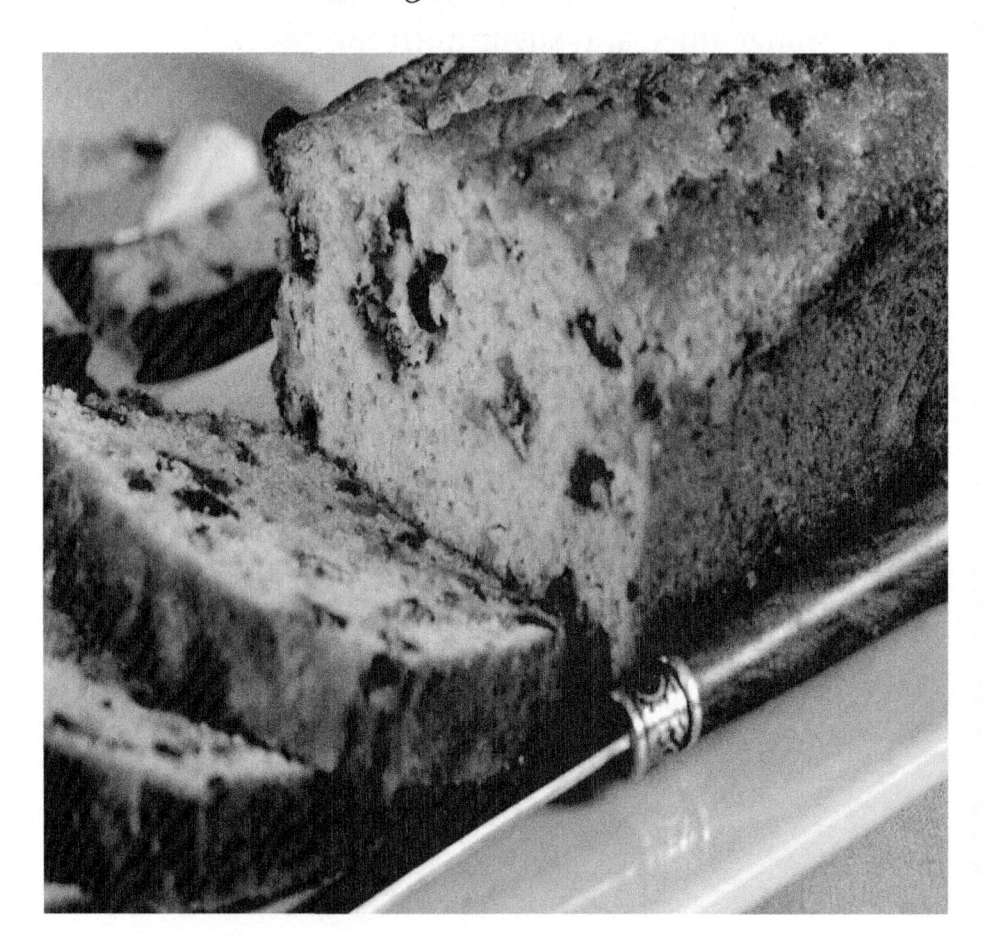

Ingredients

- 300ml (1 ¼ cups) milk, unsweetened
- 60ml (¼ cup) olive oil

- 2 egg whites
- 1 tablespoon apple cider vinegar
- ½ teaspoon baking powder
- 7g (2 teaspoons) dry active yeast
- 4 tablespoons granulated sugar
- 200g (2 cups) gluten free almond flour / or any other gluten free flour, leveled
- 100g (1 cup) Tapioca / potato starch, leveled
- 2 teaspoons Xanthan Gum
- 1 teaspoon salt
- 45g (½ cup) almonds, toasted
- 60g (½ cup) dried cranberries

Directions

- According to the manufacturer of your bread machine, into the greased pan of bread machine place all the ingredients.
- Select basic cycle / normal cycle / bake / quick bread / sweet bread setting, then select crust color either medium or light and press start to bake bread.
- In the last kneading cycle check the consistency of dough; it should be wet but thick, not like traditional bread dough. If dough is too wet, add in flour, 1 tablespoon at a time, or until dough slightly firm. If dough is too dry, add water, 1

tablespoon at a time, or until dough is slightly firm.
- When the baking cycle is finished and machine turns off, remove baked bread from pan and cool on wire rack.

Nutritional information:

150 Cal, 11 g total fat, 0 mg chol., 213 mg sodium, 5 g carb., 1 g fiber, 7 g protein.

Fruit Loaf

Yield: About 1½ Pounds loaf
Bread Machine Time: 3 hours

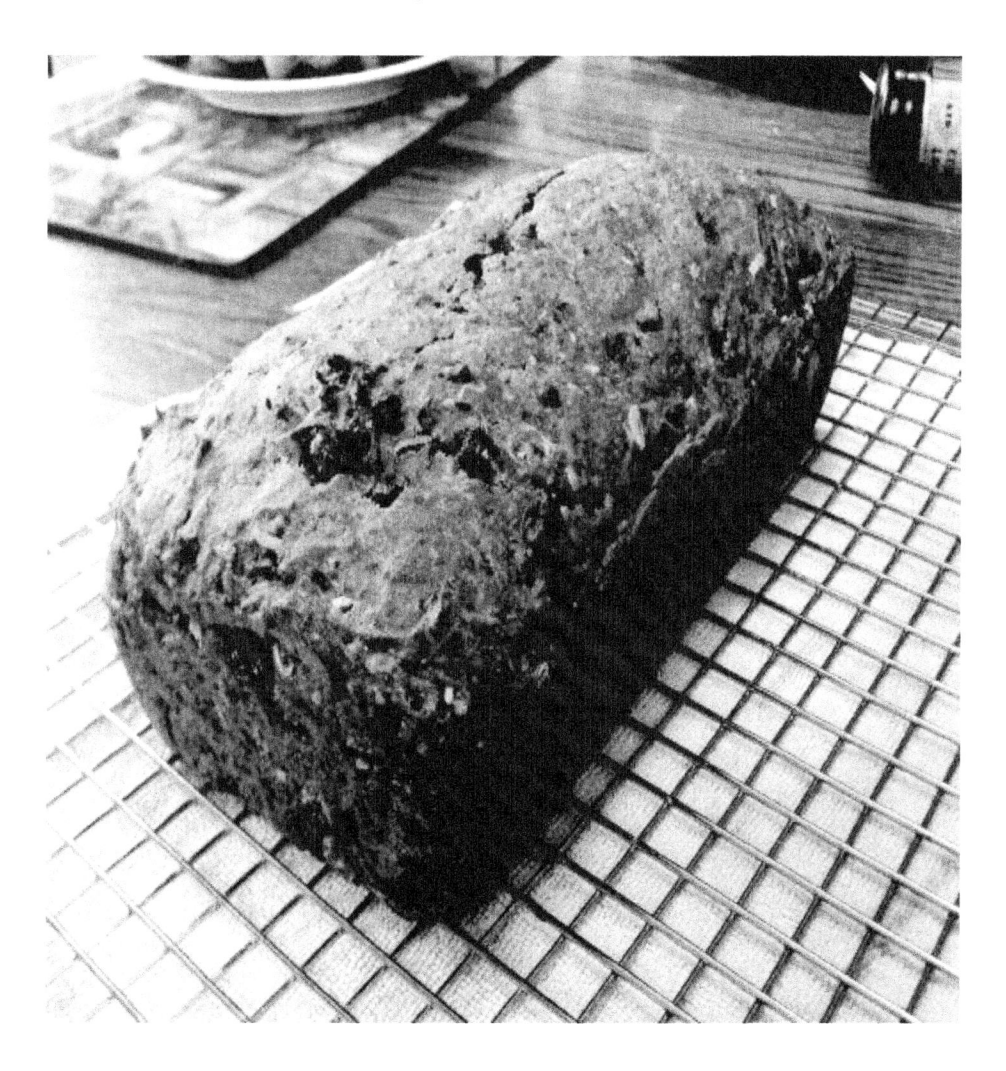

Ingredients
- 300ml (1 ¼ cups) milk, unsweetened
- 60ml (¼ cup) olive oil
- 2 egg whites
- 1 tablespoon apple cider vinegar
- ½ teaspoon baking powder
- 7g (2 teaspoons) dry active yeast
- 4 tablespoons granulated sugar
- 200g (2 cups) gluten free almond flour / or any other gluten free flour, leveled
- 100g (1 cup) Tapioca / potato starch, leveled
- 2 teaspoons Xanthan Gum
- 1 teaspoon salt
- 40g (¼ cup) dried raisins
- 38g (¼ cup) dried sultanas

Directions
- According to the manufacturer of your bread machine, into the greased pan of bread machine place all the ingredients except raisins and sultanas.
- Select basic cycle / normal cycle / bake / quick bread / sweet bread setting, then select crust color either medium or light and press start to bake bread.

- In the last kneading cycle check the consistency of dough; it should be wet but thick, not like traditional bread dough. If dough is too wet, add in flour, 1 tablespoon at a time, or until dough slightly firm. If dough is too dry, add water, 1 tablespoon at a time, or until dough is slightly firm.
- Add raisins and sultanas 5 minutes before kneading cycle ends.
- When the baking cycle is finished and machine turns off, remove baked bread from pan and cool on wire rack.
- Remove baked bread from pan and cool on wire rack.

Nutritional information:

102 Cal, 1 g total fat, 0 mg chol., 113 mg sodium, 18 g carb.,1 g fiber, 3 g protein.

Maple Syrup & Spiced Bread

Yield: About 1½ Pounds loaf
Bread Machine Time: 3 hours

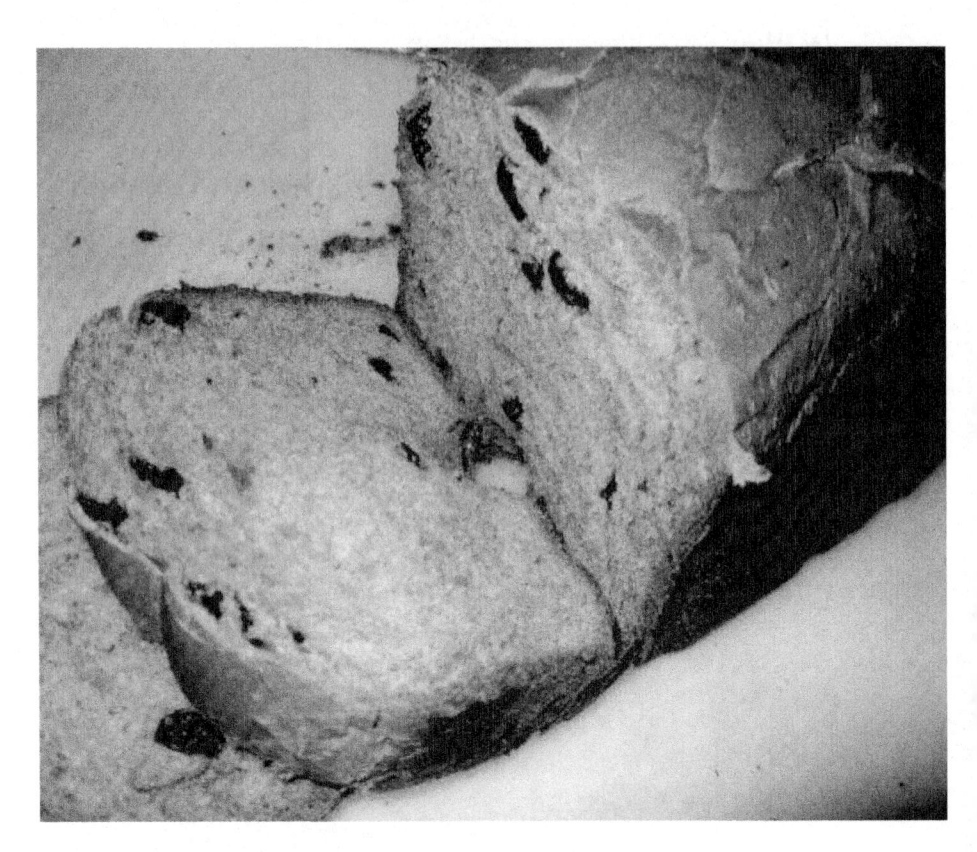

Ingredients

- 300ml (1 ¼ cups) milk, unsweetened
- ¼ cup butter, soften
- ½ tablespoons maple syrup

- 2 egg whites
- 1 tablespoon apple cider vinegar
- ½ teaspoon baking powder
- 7g (2 teaspoons) dry active yeast
- 3 tablespoons granulated sugar
- 200g (2 cups) gluten free almond flour / or any other gluten free flour, leveled
- 100g (1 cup) Tapioca / potato starch, leveled
- 2 teaspoons Xanthan Gum
- 1 teaspoon salt
- 1 tablespoon grated dried orange peel
- ½ teaspoon nutmeg
- 1 teaspoon cinnamon
- 75g (½ cup) raisins

Directions

- According to the manufacturer of your bread machine, into the greased pan of bread machine place all the ingredients.
- Select basic cycle / normal cycle / bake / quick bread / sweet bread setting, then select crust color either medium or light and press start to bake bread.
- In the last kneading cycle check the consistency of dough; it should be wet but thick, not like traditional bread dough. If dough is too wet, add in flour, 1 tablespoon at a time, or until dough slightly firm. If dough is too dry, add water, 1

tablespoon at a time, or until dough is slightly firm.
- When the baking cycle is finished and machine turns off, remove baked bread from pan and cool on wire rack.

Nutritional information:

186 Cal, 8 g total fat, 0 mg chol., 150 mg sodium, 24 g carb., 1 g fiber, 4 g protein.

Peanut Butter & Jelly Bread

Yield: About 1½ Pounds loaf
Bread Machine Time: 3 hours

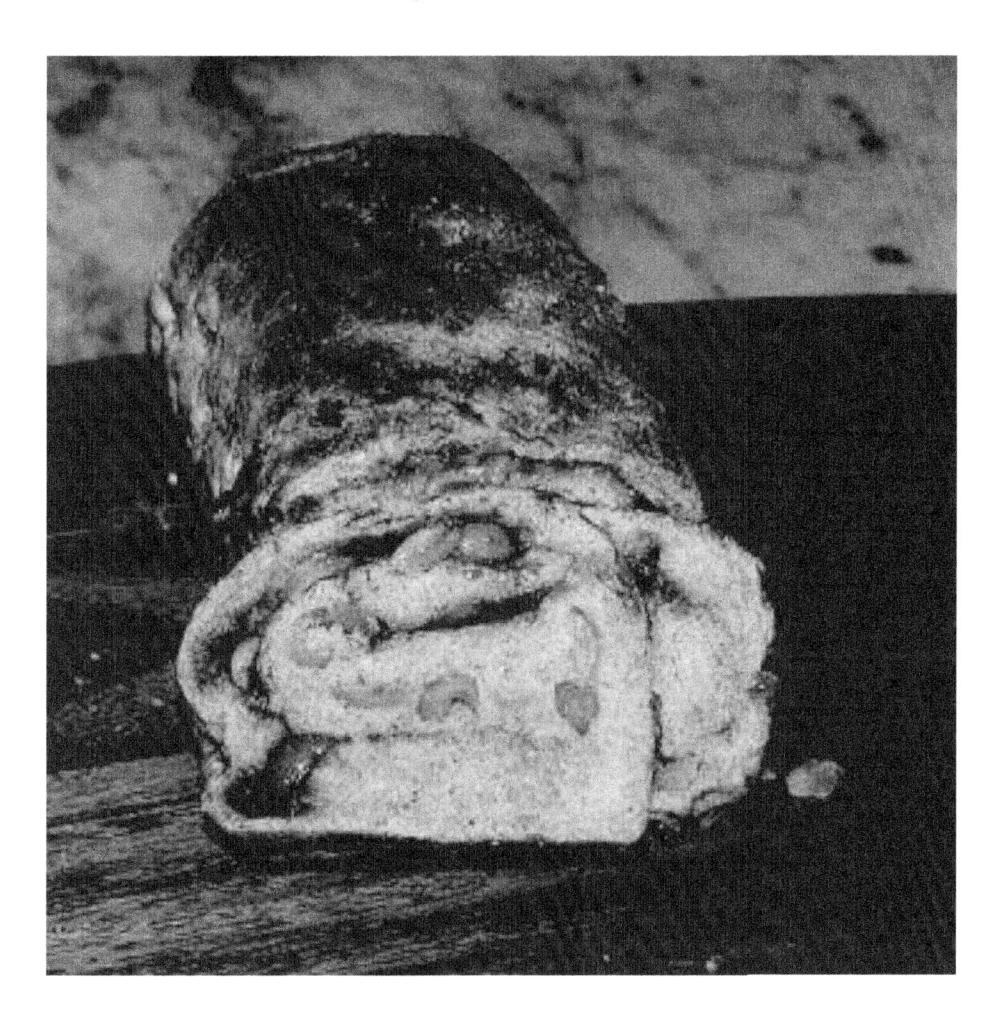

Ingredients
- 300ml (1 ¼ cups) water
- 2 tablespoons olive oil
- 115g (½ cup) unsalted dry-roasted peanuts
- 7g (2 teaspoons) dry active yeast
- 2 tablespoons granulated sugar
- 200g (2 cups) gluten free almond flour / or any other gluten free flour, leveled
- 100g (1 cup) Tapioca / potato starch, leveled
- 2 teaspoons Xanthan Gum
- 1 teaspoon salt
- ½ teaspoon baking powder
- 1 tablespoon apple cider vinegar
- 2 egg whites
- 108g (½ cup) jelly

Directions
- According to the manufacturer of your bread machine, into the greased pan of bread machine place all the ingredients.
- Select basic cycle / normal cycle / bake / quick bread / sweet bread setting, then select crust color either medium or light and press start to bake bread.
- In the last kneading cycle check the consistency of dough; it should be wet but thick, not like

traditional bread dough. If dough is too wet, add in flour, 1 tablespoon at a time, or until dough slightly firm. If dough is too dry, add water, 1 tablespoon at a time, or until dough is slightly firm.
- When the baking cycle is finished and machine turns off, remove baked bread from pan and cool on wire rack.

Nutritional information:

225 Cal, 15 g total fat, 0 mg chol., 115 mg sodium, 34 g carb., 7 g fiber, 12 g protein.

Gluten free bread rolls & buns

Pizza Crust

Yield: About 2 crusts
Preparation Time: 2 hours and 15 minutes
Baking Time: 45 minutes

Ingredients

- 237ml (1 cup) warm milk
- 5 egg whites
- 60ml (¼ cup) olive oil
- 1 tablespoon apple cider vinegar
- ½ teaspoon baking powder
- 7g (2 teaspoons) dry active yeast
- 2 tablespoons granulated sugar
- 200g (2 cups) gluten free almond flour / or any other gluten free flour, leveled
- 100g (1 cup) Tapioca / potato starch, leveled
- 2 teaspoons Xanthan Gum
- 1 teaspoon salt

Directions

- According to the manufacturer of your bread machine, into the greased pan of bread machine

place all the ingredients, select dough / knead / manual cycle to prepare dough and press start.
- In the meantime, grease two medium sized pizza pans and set aside until require.
- When kneading cycle ends, using floured hands transfer dough onto a clean working space, dusted with flour. Punch down dough, knead for 4-5 times and divide into half.
- Shape each half into round and using rolling pin, roll into crust according to desire thickness. Roll each crust around rolling pin and unroll on each pizza pan. Cover each pan with damp towel and let rest for 45-60 minutes or until doubles in size.
- When the dough risen either store in freezer or decorate with favorite toppings to bake straightaway in a preheated oven at 350 degrees F for 45 minutes.

Nutritional information:

130 Cal, 2g total fat, 0 mg chol., 240 mg sodium, 24 g carb., 3 g fiber, 4 g protein.

Italian Bread

Yield: About 2 loaves
Preparation Time: 2 hours and 30 minutes
Baking Time: 45 minutes

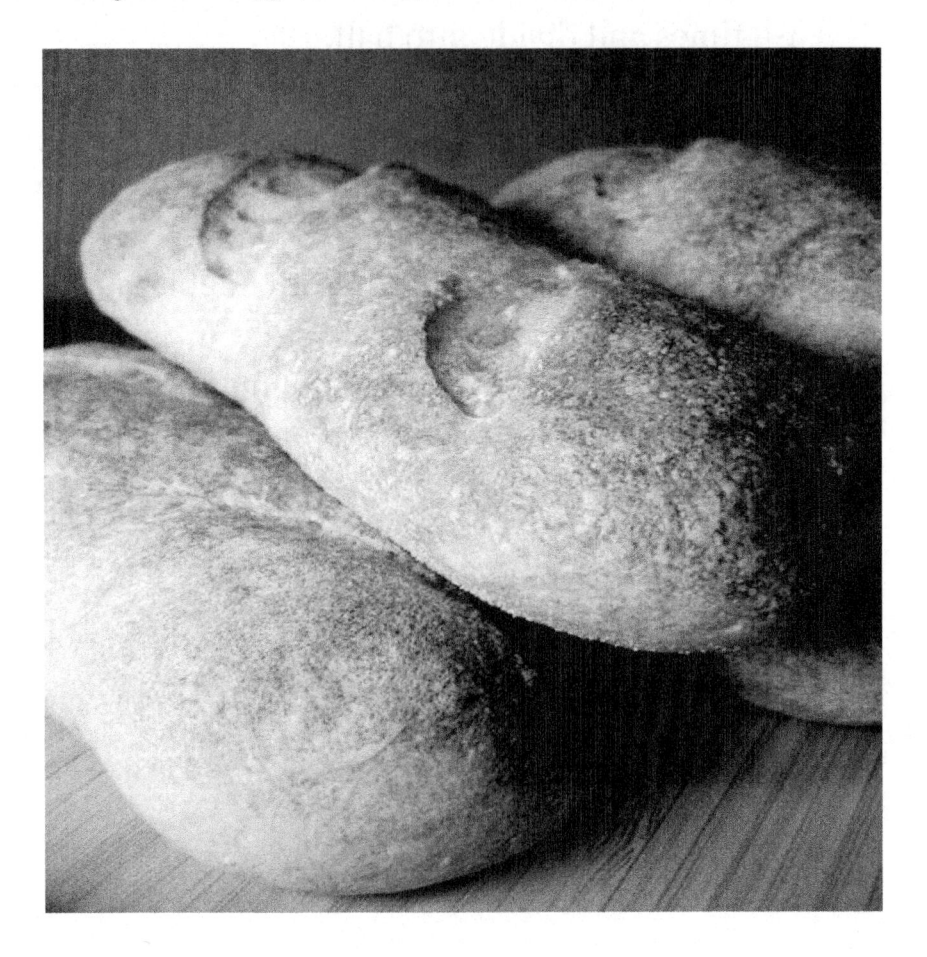

Ingredients
- 237ml (1 cup) warm water

- 3 egg whites, divided
- 60ml (¼ cup) olive oil
- 1 tablespoon apple cider vinegar
- ½ teaspoon baking powder
- 7g (2 teaspoons) dry active yeast
- 1 tablespoon granulated sugar
- 200g (2 cups) gluten free almond flour / or any other gluten free flour, leveled
- 100g (1 cup) Tapioca / potato starch, leveled
- 2 teaspoons Xanthan Gum
- 1 teaspoon salt
- 2 tablespoons cornmeal

Directions

- According to the manufacturer of your bread machine, into the greased pan of bread machine place all the ingredients except reserving one egg white and cornmeal.
- Select dough / knead / manual cycle to prepare dough and press start.
- When kneading cycle ends, using floured hands transfer dough onto a clean working space, dusted with flour. Punch down dough and shape evenly into two loaves. Generously sprinkle cornmeal over loaves, then cover with a damp towel and let rest for 30-45 minutes or until dough doubles in size.

- While loaves rises, place baking rack in the middle of oven, set temperature at 375 degrees F and let preheat. Grease a large baking tray and set aside until require.
- In a bowl beat reserve egg white with 1 tablespoon water or until combine.
- Brush risen loaves with egg mixture and using a sharp knife make a long cut down the center of loaves and then slide loaves carefully in one quick motion onto a prepared baking tray.
- Bake loaves for 30-45 minutes until crust is nicely golden brown and when tap on the bottom, loaves should sound hollow.
- Transfer baked loaves onto wire rack and let cool before serving.

Nutritional information:

91 Cal, 9 g total fat, 0 mg chol., 175 mg sodium, 15 g carb., 1 g fiber, 3 g protein.

Hot Cross Buns

Yield: About 12 buns
Preparation Time: 2 hours and 10 minutes
Baking Time: 25 minutes

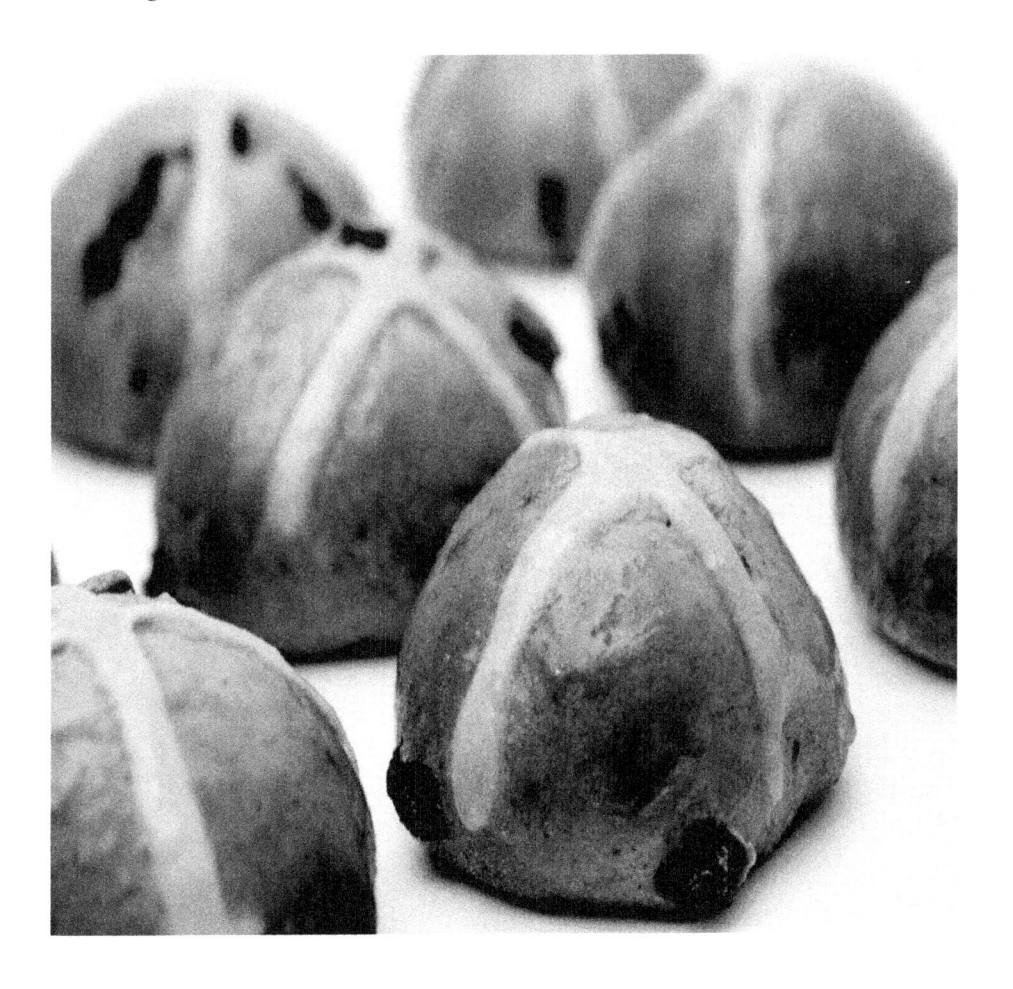

Ingredients
For the bread

- 178ml (¾ cup) warm milk
- 3 tablespoons fat-free butter, unsalted
- 4 egg whites, divided
- 1 tablespoon apple cider vinegar
- ½ teaspoon baking powder
- 7g (2 teaspoons) dry active yeast
- 3 tablespoons granulated sugar
- 200g (2 cups) gluten free almond flour / or any other gluten free flour, leveled
- 100g (1 cup) Tapioca / potato starch, leveled
- 2 teaspoons Xanthan Gum
- ½ teaspoon salt
- 1 teaspoon ground cinnamon
- 115g (¾ cup) dried currants

For the glaze

- ½ cup confectioners' sugar
- ¼ teaspoon vanilla extract

Directions
- According to the manufacturer of your bread machine, into the greased pan of bread machine

place all the ingredients except cinnamon and currants and reserve 1 egg white.
- Select dough / knead / manual cycle to prepare dough and press start. Add cinnamon and currants 5 minutes before kneading cycle ends.
- When kneading cycle ends, using floured hands transfer dough onto a clean working space, dusted with flour.
- Punch down dough, cover with a damp towel and let rest for 15 minutes. Then shape dough evenly into 12 balls and arrange in a greased 9 by 13 inch baking sheet. Cover pan with a damp towel and let rest in a warm place for 30-45 minutes until double in size.
- In the meantime, place baking rack in the middle of oven, set temperature at 375 degrees F and let preheat.
- In a bowl beat reserve egg white with 1 tablespoon water or until combine.
- Place raised buns sheet into oven and bake for 20-25 minutes or until nicely golden brown and inserted wooden skewer into the center of buns come out clean.
- While buns bake, in a bowl combine confectioners' sugar, vanilla and 2 tablespoons milk until mix well.
- Transfer baked buns onto a wire rack and let cool completely. Make an X on each bun using vanilla-sugar mixture and serve.

Nutritional information:

111 Cal, 5 g total fat, 0 mg chol., 101 mg sodium, 19 g carb., 1 g fiber, 3 g protein.

Bread Sticks

Yield: About 18 breadsticks
Preparation Time: 1 hour
Baking Time: 20 minutes

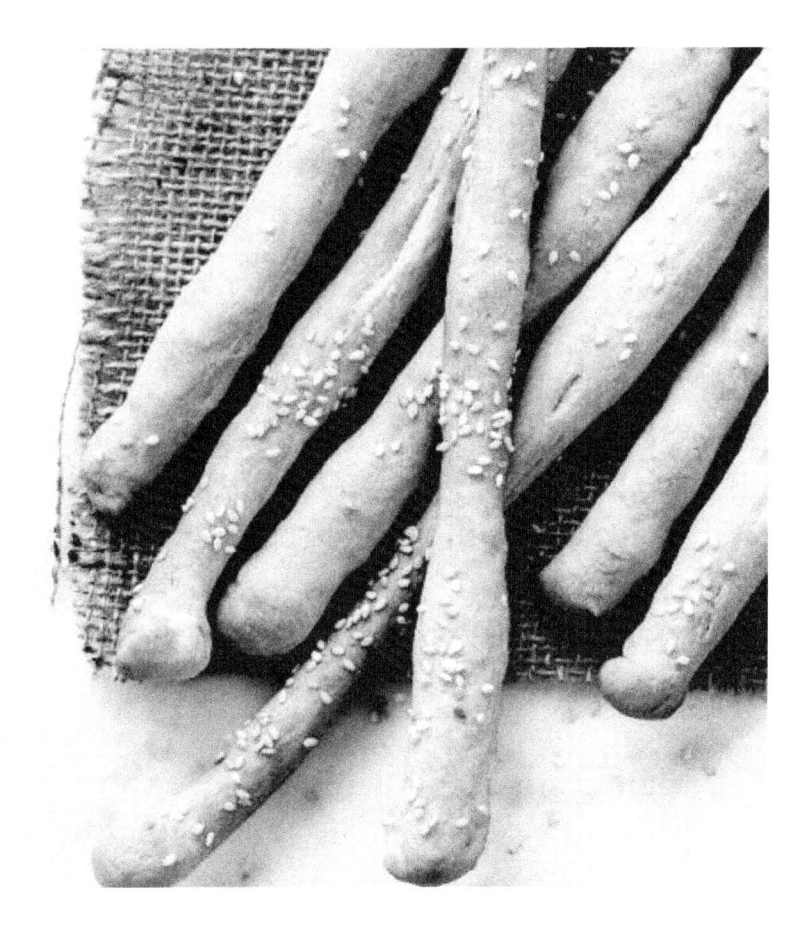

Ingredients
- 237ml (1 cups) warm milk

- 3 tablespoons fat-free butter, unsalted
- 2 egg whites
- 1 tablespoon apple cider vinegar
- ½ teaspoon baking powder
- 7g (2 teaspoons) dry active yeast
- 2 tablespoons granulated sugar
- 200g (2 cups) gluten free almond flour / or any other gluten free flour, leveled
- 100g (1 cup) Tapioca / potato starch, leveled
- 2 teaspoons Xanthan Gum
- 1 teaspoon salt
- 3 tablespoons sesame seeds

Directions

- According to the manufacturer of your bread machine, into the greased pan of bread machine place all the ingredients.
- Select dough / knead / manual cycle to prepare dough and press start.
- When kneading cycle ends, using floured hands transfer dough onto a clean working space, lightly greased with oil.
- Place baking rack in the middle of oven, set temperature at 375 degrees F and let preheat. Lightly grease two 9 by 13 inch baking sheets.
- Punch down dough and divide evenly into 18 pieces. Roll each piece and form breadstick by rolling from the center to the outside edges.

- Arrange breadsticks into prepared baking sheets, 1 inch apart, and place into the oven.
- Bake for 15-20 minutes until crust is nicely golden brown, switch sheets position halfway through baking.
- Remove breadsticks to cooling racks and cool completely before serving.

Nutritional information:

84 Cal, 2 g total fat, 0 mg chol., 93 mg sodium, 12.13 g carb., 1 g fiber, 2 g protein.

Cinnamon Buns

Yield: About 8 buns
Preparation Time: 2 hours
Baking Time: 25 minutes

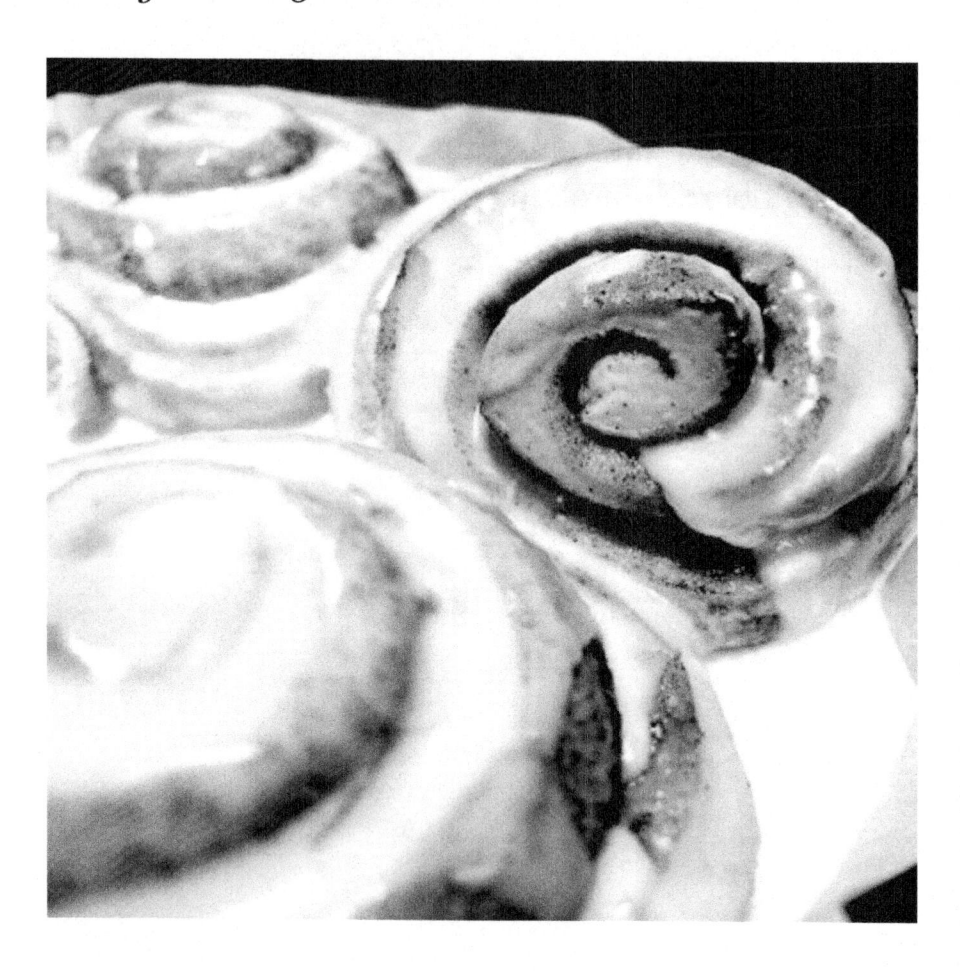

Ingredients
For the bread

- 300ml (1 ¼ cups) milk, unsweetened
- 3 egg whites, divided
- 1 tablespoon apple cider vinegar
- ½ teaspoon baking powder
- 7g (2 teaspoons) dry active yeast
- 2 tablespoons granulated sugar
- 4 tablespoons melted fat-free butter, unsalted
- 200g (2 cups) gluten free almond flour / or any other gluten free flour, leveled
- 100g (1 cup) Tapioca / potato starch, leveled
- 2 teaspoons Xanthan Gum
- 50g (½ cup) instant vanilla pudding mix
- 1 teaspoon salt
- 115g (½ cup) soften fat-free butter, unsalted
- 165g (¾ cup) packed brown sugar
- 1 teaspoon ground cinnamon
- 2 tablespoons walnuts
- 2 tablespoons raisins

For the glaze

- 63g (½ cup) confectioners' sugar
- ¼ teaspoon vanilla extract
- 4 tablespoons soften fat-free butter, unsalted

- 1 teaspoon milk

Directions
- According to the manufacturer of your bread machine, into the greased pan of bread machine place all the ingredients except butter, brown sugar, cinnamon, walnuts and raisins.
- Select dough / knead / manual cycle to prepare dough and press start.
- When kneading cycle ends, using floured hands transfer dough onto a clean working space, dusted with flour. Punch down dough, knead 4-5 times and then using rolling pin shape dough into a large rectangle.
- In a small bowl stir together butter, brown sugar and cinnamon until combine and then spread evenly over the dough. Sprinkle with chopped walnuts and raisins and then roll dough into a log, starting from the widest edge.
- Seal seams by pinching dough, then cut dough into 1 inch slices and arrange onto the prepared pan, 1 inch apart. Cover pan and let rest for 30-45 minutes in a warm place or until doubles in size.
- In the meantime, place baking rack in the middle of oven, set temperature at 350 degrees F and let preheat. Lightly grease 9 by 13 inch baking sheet.
- Place baking sheet into oven and bake for 20-25 minutes or until nicely golden brown.

- While buns cool, prepare glaze. In a bowl stir together confectioners' sugar, vanilla, butter and milk until combine.
- Transfer baked buns onto cooling rack, let cool for 10 minutes. Spread prepared glaze over buns and serve immediately.

Nutritional information:

145 Cal, 5 g total fat, 0 mg chol., 340 mg sodium, 23 g carb., 1 g fiber, 2 g protein.

Burger Buns

Yield: About 12 buns
Preparation Time: 2 hours and 10 minutes
Baking Time: 12 minutes

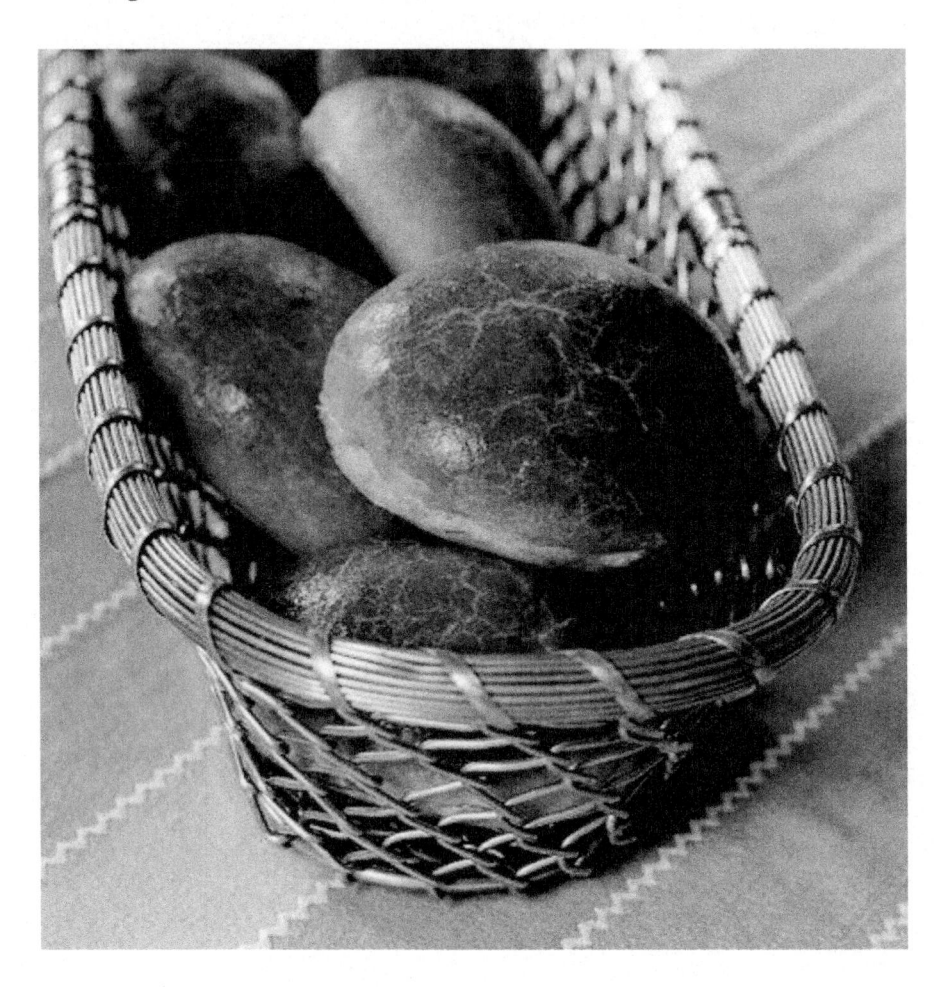

Ingredients
- 300ml (1 ¼ cups) warm milk
- 60ml (¼ cup) olive oil
- 4 tablespoons melted fat-free butter, unsalted
- 3 egg whites
- 1 tablespoon apple cider vinegar
- ½ teaspoon baking powder
- 7g (2 teaspoons) dry active yeast
- 4 tablespoons granulated sugar
- 200g (2 cups) gluten free almond flour / or any other gluten free flour, leveled
- 100g (1 cup) Tapioca / potato starch, leveled
- 2 teaspoons Xanthan Gum
- ½ teaspoon salt

Directions
- According to the manufacturer of your bread machine, into the greased pan of bread machine place all the ingredients except butter.
- Select dough / knead / manual cycle to prepare dough and press start.
- When kneading cycle ends, using floured hands transfer dough onto a clean working space, dusted with flour. Punch down dough, knead for 4-5 times, shape into a round and cut evenly into two halves.

- Working on one half at a time, roll a half into 1 inch thick round and then using inverted glass as a cutter cut out six rounds, each 3 ½ inch diameter.
- Cut out more six round from the other half in the same manner.
- Grease a 9 by 13 inch baking sheet, arrange buns, brush with butter, then cover with a damp towel and let rest in a warm place for 45-60 minutes until buns doubles in size.
- In the meantime, place baking rack in the middle of oven, set temperature at 350 degrees F and let preheat.
- Place baking sheet into oven and bake buns for 10-12 minutes or until crust is nicely golden brown and when tap bun should sound hollow.

Nutritional information:

130 Cal, 2 g total fat, 0 mg chol., 220 mg sodium, 23 g carb., 1 g fiber, 4 g protein.

Naan Bread

Yield: About 6 breads
Preparation Time: 1 hour and 15 minutes
Baking Time: 12 minutes

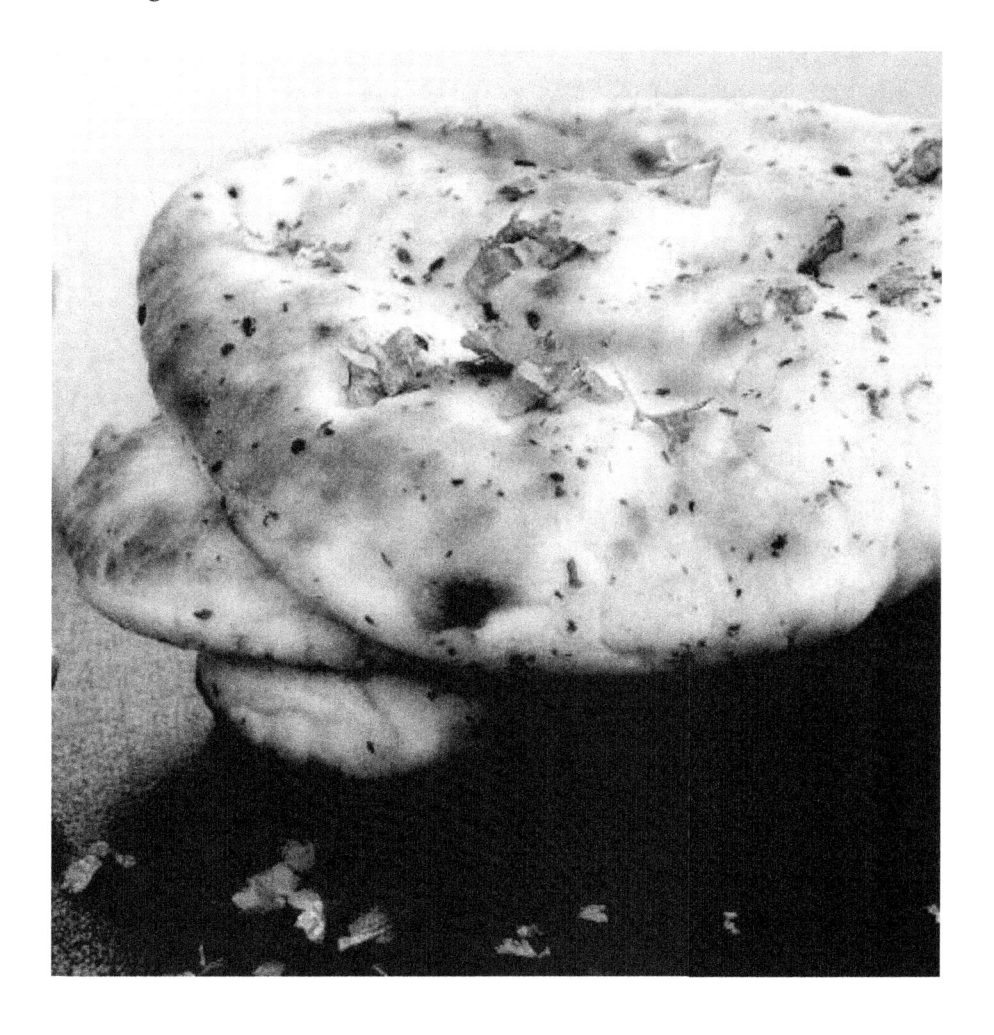

Ingredients

- 2/3 cup warm milk, unsweetened
- 2 tablespoons olive oil
- 164g (2/3 cup) low-fat yogurt
- 3 egg whites
- 1 tablespoon apple cider vinegar
- ½ teaspoon baking powder
- 7g (2 teaspoons) dry active yeast
- 2 tablespoons granulated sugar
- 2 teaspoons melted fat-free butter, unsalted
- 200g (2 cups) gluten free almond flour / or any other gluten free flour, leveled
- 100g (1 cup) Tapioca / potato starch, leveled
- 2 teaspoons Xanthan Gum
- 1 teaspoon salt

Directions

- According to the manufacturer of your bread machine, into the greased pan of bread machine place all the ingredients, select dough / knead / manual cycle to prepare dough and press start.
- When kneading cycle ends, using floured hands transfer dough onto a clean working space, dusted with flour.
- Place baking rack in the top shelf of oven, set temperature at 500 degrees F and let preheat.

- Punch down dough, knead 4-5 times and then evenly divide dough into six pieces and then shape into rounds.
- Working on each piece at a time, using rolling pin flatten dough to 1/3 inch thickness.
- Arrange one dough onto a heavy baking sheet and place into oven and bake for 90 seconds or until bread start to puff. Then switch oven to broil and broil bread for 1 minute or until nicely golden brown. Bake remaining bread in the same manner and keep warm.
- Brush each naan bread with butter and serve immediately.

Nutritional information:

137 Cal, 5 g total fat, 13 mg chol., 142 mg sodium, 19 g carb., 1 g fiber, 4 g protein.

Tomato Foccacia

Yield: About 1 loaf
Preparation Time: 2 hours
Baking Time: 20 minutes

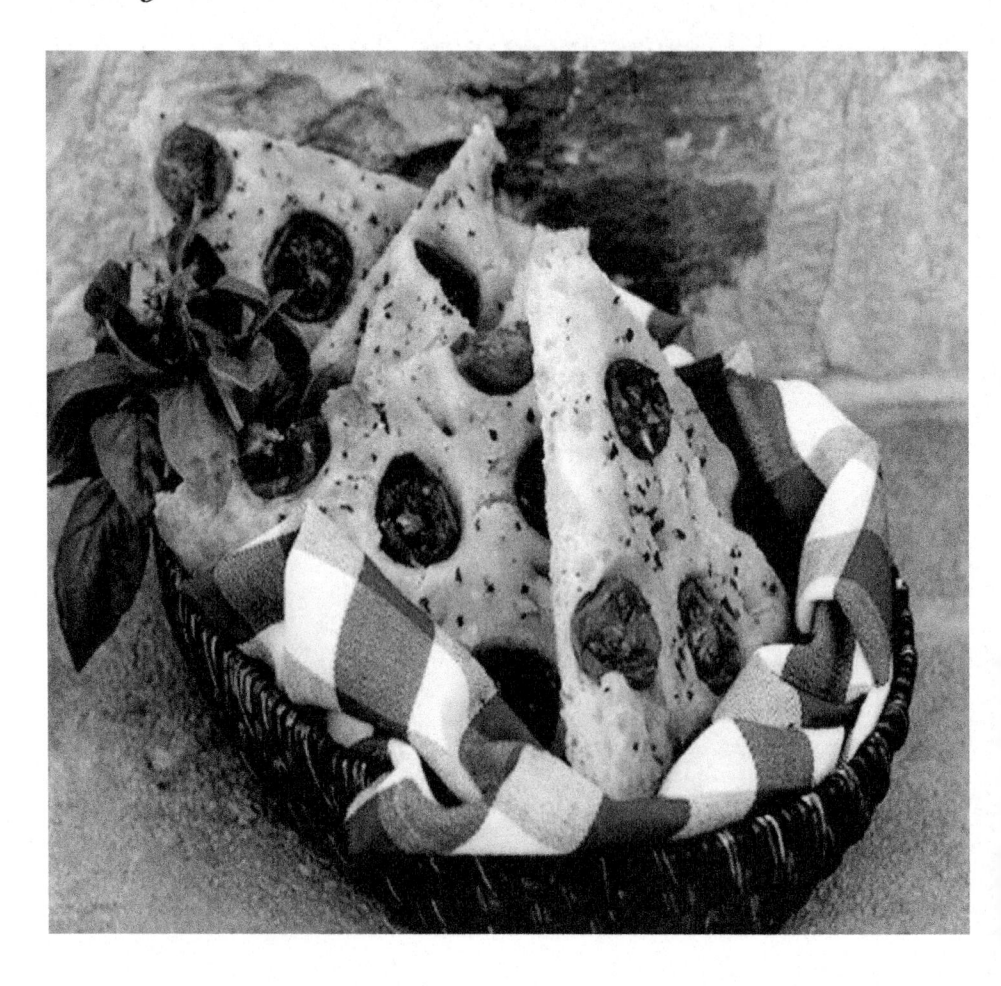

Ingredients
- 237ml (1 cup) warm milk
- 3 tablespoons soften fat-free butter, unsalted
- 3 egg whites
- 1 tablespoon apple cider vinegar
- ½ teaspoon baking powder
- 7g (2 teaspoons) dry active yeast
- 2 tablespoons granulated sugar
- 2 tablespoons olive oil
- 200g (2 cups) gluten free almond flour / or any other gluten free flour, leveled
- 100g (1 cup) Tapioca / potato starch, leveled
- 2 teaspoons Xanthan Gum
- 100g (½ cup) chopped sun-dried tomatoes
- 1 teaspoon salt
- 2 tablespoons grated Parmesan cheese
- 2 teaspoons dried rosemary, crushed
- 113g (1 cup) shredded fat-free mozzarella cheese

Directions
- According to the manufacturer of your bread machine, into the greased pan of bread machine place all the ingredients except cheeses and rosemary.
- Select dough / knead / manual cycle to prepare dough and press start.

- When kneading cycle ends, using floured hands transfer dough onto a clean working space, dusted with flour.
- Place baking rack in the middle shelf of oven, set temperature at 400 degrees F and let preheat.
- Punch down dough, knead 4-5 times, shape into a round and place dough in a greased bowl. Coat dough with oil on all sides, cover bowl with a damp towel and let rest in a warm for 15 minutes or until rise.
- Sprinkle the bottom of a medium sized baking pan with cornmeal, place risen dough and using fingers flat dough to fit the pan and make indentations with finger tips.
- Brush top with oil, cover pan with damp towel and let rest in a warm place for 30-45 minutes or until doubles in size.
- Then sprinkle cheese and rosemary over the dough and place pan into the oven.
- Bake bread for 15-20 minutes until crust is nicely golden brown and cheese melt.
- Transfer baked bread onto a cooling rack, cool for 10 minutes and then slice to serve.

Nutritional information:

110 Cal, 3 g total fat, 0 mg chol., 200 mg sodium, 18 g carb., 1 g fiber, 4 g protein.

Challah Bread

Yield: About 2 loaves
Preparation Time: 1 hour and 45 minutes
Baking Time: 35 minutes

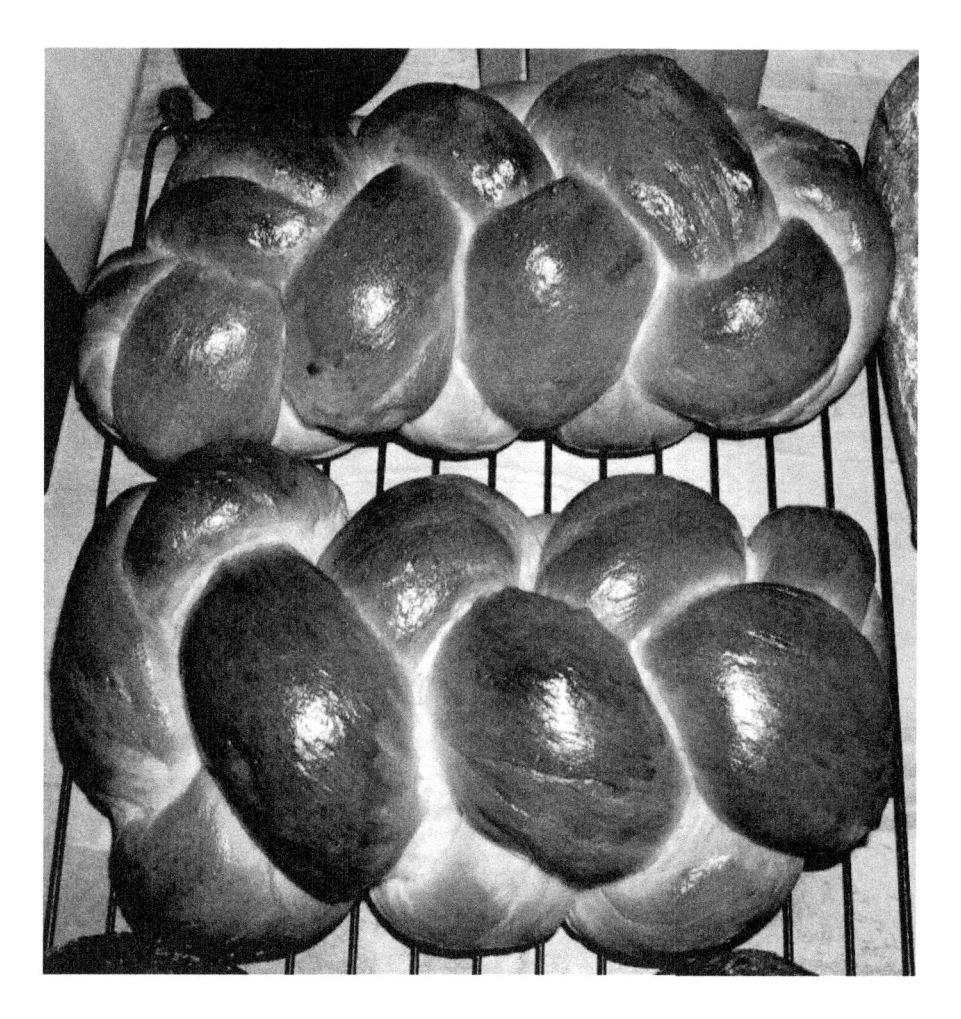

Ingredients
- 300ml (1 ¼ cups) warm water
- 60ml (¼ cup) olive oil
- 1 tablespoon apple cider vinegar
- ½ teaspoon baking powder
- 7g (2 teaspoons) dry active yeast
- 2 tablespoons granulated sugar
- 200g (2 cups) gluten free almond flour / or any other gluten free flour, leveled
- 100g (1 cup) Tapioca / potato starch, leveled
- 2 teaspoons Xanthan Gum
- 1 teaspoon salt
- 4 egg whites, divided
- 1 tablespoon poppy seeds
- 1 tablespoon sesame seeds

Directions
- According to the manufacturer of your bread machine, into the greased pan of bread machine place all the ingredients except poppy seeds and reserve 1 week.
- Select dough / knead / manual cycle to prepare dough and press start.
- When kneading cycle ends, using floured hands transfer dough onto a clean working space, dusted with flour.

- Place baking rack in the middle shelf of oven, set temperature at 350 degrees F and let preheat.
- Punch down dough, knead for 4-5 times and then divide dough into half. Divide each half further into three pieces and roll piece into long log.
- Prepare challah bread. First pinch together the top of three logs, then braid three logs and then pinch the bottom ends. Prepare second challah bread with remaining three logs in the same manner.
- Grease a 9 by 13 inch baking sheet, arrange both challah breads, cover pan with dampen towel and let rest in a warm place for 30-45 minutes or until doubles in size.
- In a bowl beat reserve egg white with 1 tablespoon water and then brush over raised challah breads.
- Sprinkle evenly with sesame seeds and poppy seeds and bake breads for 30-35 minutes or until crust is evenly golden brown.
- Transfer baked breads onto cooling rack and cool completely before serving.

Nutritional information:

90 Cal, 3g total fat, 0 mg chol., 63 mg sodium, 15g carb., 1 g fiber, 3 g protein.

Sweet Dinner Rolls

Yield: About 16 rolls
Preparation Time: 2 hours
Baking Time: 20 minutes

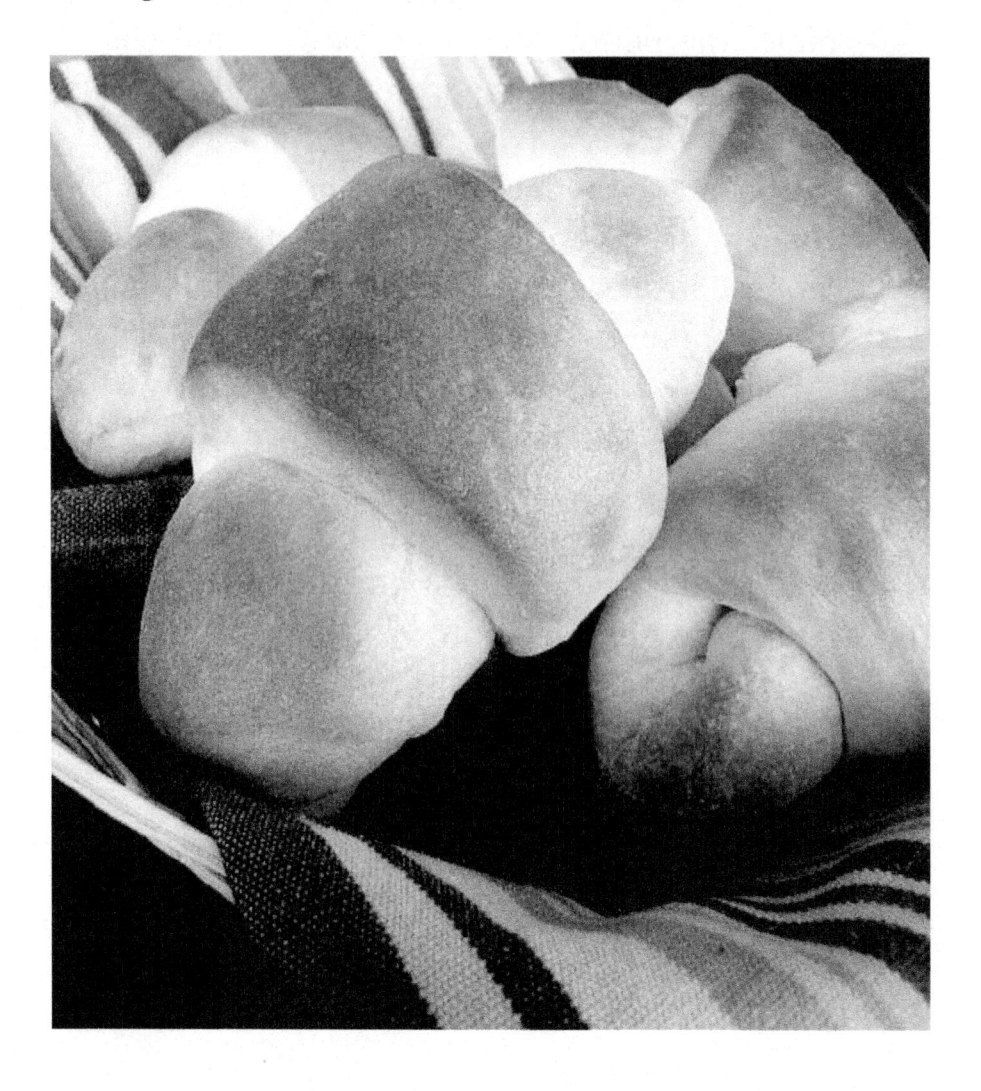

114

Ingredients
- 1 cup warm milk
- 3 egg whites
- 1 tablespoon apple cider vinegar
- ½ teaspoon baking powder
- 7g (2 teaspoons) dry active yeast
- 2 tablespoons granulated sugar
- 58g (¼ cup) soften fat-free butter, unsalted, & more as needed
- 200g (2 cups) gluten free almond flour / or any other gluten free flour, leveled
- 100g (1 cup) Tapioca / potato starch, leveled
- 2 teaspoons Xanthan Gum
- 1 teaspoon salt

Directions
- According to the manufacturer of your bread machine, into the greased pan of bread machine place all the ingredients, select dough / knead / manual cycle to prepare dough and press start.
- When kneading cycle ends, using floured hands transfer dough onto a clean working space, dusted with flour. Punch down dough, knead 4-5 times and divide into half.
- Work on one dough-half at a time. Shape one half into 12 inch diameter round, spread ¼ cup butter over the entire dough and then cut into 8

wedges. Cut more 8 wedges from the other half in the same manner.
- Roll each wedge tightly, starting from wide end and then arrange on a ungreased 9 by 13 inch baking sheet, point side down. Cover pan with damp towel and let rest in a warm place for 1 hour or until doubles in size.
- In the meantime, place baking rack in the middle shelf of oven, set temperature at 375 degrees F and let preheat.
- Place baking sheet into oven and bake for 15-20 minutes or until nicely golden brown.
- Transfer baked bread rolls onto cooling rack and cool completely before serving.

Nutritional information:

88 Cal, 2 g total fat, 1 mg chol., 134 mg sodium, 13 g carb., 1 g fiber, 3 g protein.

French Baguettes

Yield: About 2 loaves
Preparation Time: 2 hours and 30 minutes
Baking Time: 25 minutes

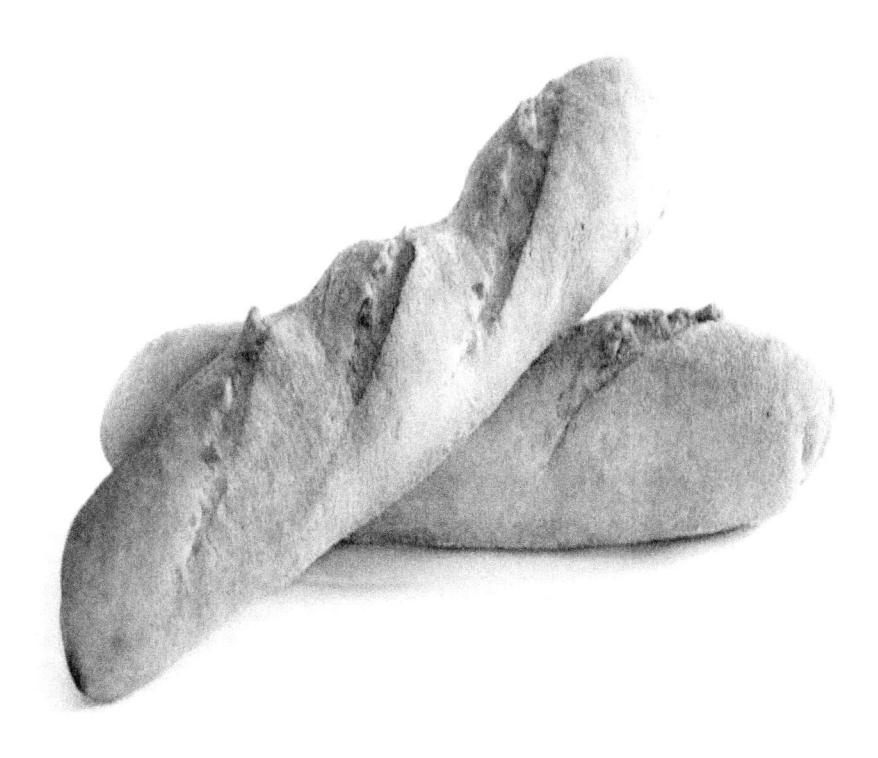

Ingredients
- 300ml (1 ¼ cups) warm water
- 60ml (¼ cup) olive oil
- 1 tablespoon apple cider vinegar
- ½ teaspoon baking powder
- 7g (2 teaspoons) dry active yeast
- 2 tablespoons granulated sugar
- 200g (2 cups) gluten free almond flour / or any other gluten free flour, leveled
- 100g (1 cup) Tapioca / potato starch, leveled
- 2 teaspoons Xanthan Gum
- 1 teaspoon salt
- 3 egg whites, divided

Directions
- According to the manufacturer of your bread machine, into the greased pan of bread machine place all the ingredients, reserve 1 egg white.
- Select dough / knead / manual cycle to prepare dough and press start.
- When kneading cycle ends, using floured hands transfer dough onto a clean working space, dusted with flour. Punch down dough, knead for 4-5 times and place into a greased bowl.
- Brush oil all over the dough, cover with dampen towel and let rest in a warm place for 30-45 minutes or until doubles in size.

- Transfer raised dough onto lightly floured working space, punch dough and then roll dough into a rectangle. Then dough into half, creating two rectangles, and then tightly roll each half starting from wide edge.
- Grease a 9 by 15 inch baking sheet and place rolls, 3 inch apart. Using a sharp knife make one cut lengthwise on each loaf. Cover pan with a damp towel and let rest in a warm place for 30-45 minutes or until double in size.
- In the meantime, place baking rack in the top shelf of oven, set temperature at 375 degrees F and let preheat.
- In a bowl beat together reserve egg white with 1 tablespoon water until combine.
- Spread beaten egg mixture generously over raised loaves and then place baking sheet into oven to bake for 20-25 minutes or until evenly golden brown.
- Removed baked loaves to cooling rack and let cool before serving.

Nutritional information:

150 Cal, 9 g total fat, 0 mg chol., 370 mg sodium, 30 g carb., 1 g fiber, 5 g protein.

Onion Sandwich Rolls

Yield: About 8 rolls
Preparation Time: 1 hour and 45 minutes
Baking Time: 25 minutes

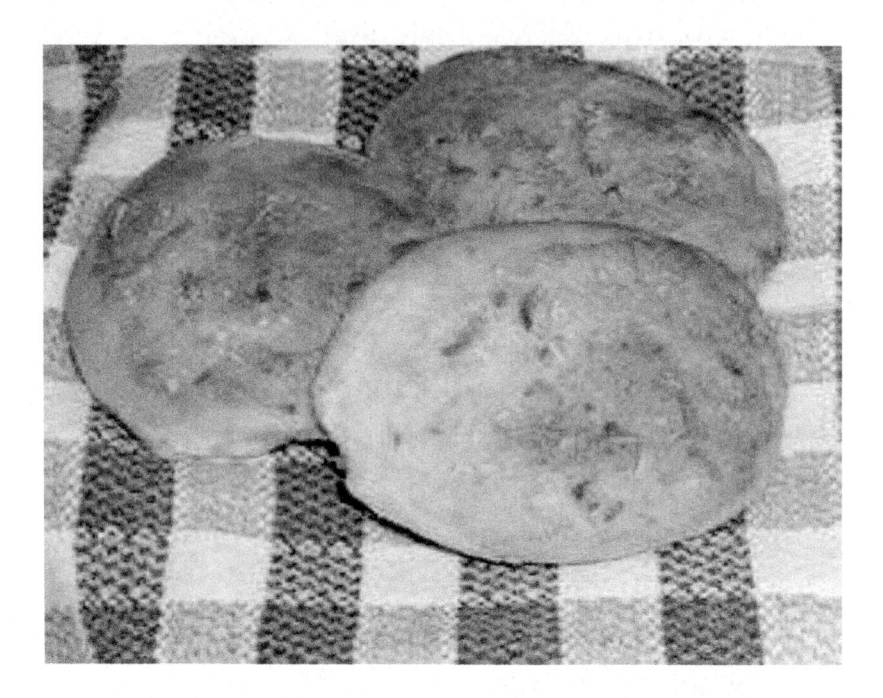

Ingredients
- 1 ¼ cups warm milk
- 3 egg whites, divided
- 3 tablespoons soften fat-free butter, unsalted
- 1 tablespoon apple cider vinegar
- ½ teaspoon baking powder
- 7g (2 teaspoons) dry active yeast

- 2 tablespoons granulated sugar
- 1 teaspoon onion powder
- 200g (2 cups) gluten free almond flour / or any other gluten free flour, leveled
- 100g (1 cup) Tapioca / potato starch, leveled
- 2 teaspoons Xanthan Gum
- 3 tablespoons dried minced onion & more as needed
- 45g (¼ cup) instant potato flakes
- 1 teaspoon salt

Directions

- According to the manufacturer of your bread machine, into the greased pan of bread machine place all the ingredients, reserve 1 egg white.
- Select dough / knead / manual cycle to prepare dough and press start.
- When kneading cycle ends, using floured hands transfer dough onto a clean working space, dusted with flour. Punch down dough, knead for 4-5 times, divide evenly into 8 pieces and shape each piece into ball.
- Using rolling pin, flat each ball into 4 inch diameter crust and place on a large baking sheet. Cover pan with a damp towel and let rest in a warm place for 30-45 minutes or until double in size.

- In the meantime, place baking rack in the top shelf of oven, set temperature at 350 degrees F and let preheat.
- In a bowl beat reserve egg white and 1 tablespoon water until combine and brush over each raised crust.
- Sprinkle with dried minced onion and place baking sheet into the oven to bake for 20-25 minutes until nicely golden brown.
- Transfer bake breads onto cooling rack and cool completely.
- Slice each bread horizontally before serving.

Nutritional information:

150 Cal, 3g total fat, 0 mg chol., 230 mg sodium, 28 g carb., 1 g fiber, 6 g protein.

<u>Hawaiian Bread Rolls</u>

Yield: About 12 rolls
Preparation Time: 1 hour and 45 minutes
Baking Time: 25 minutes

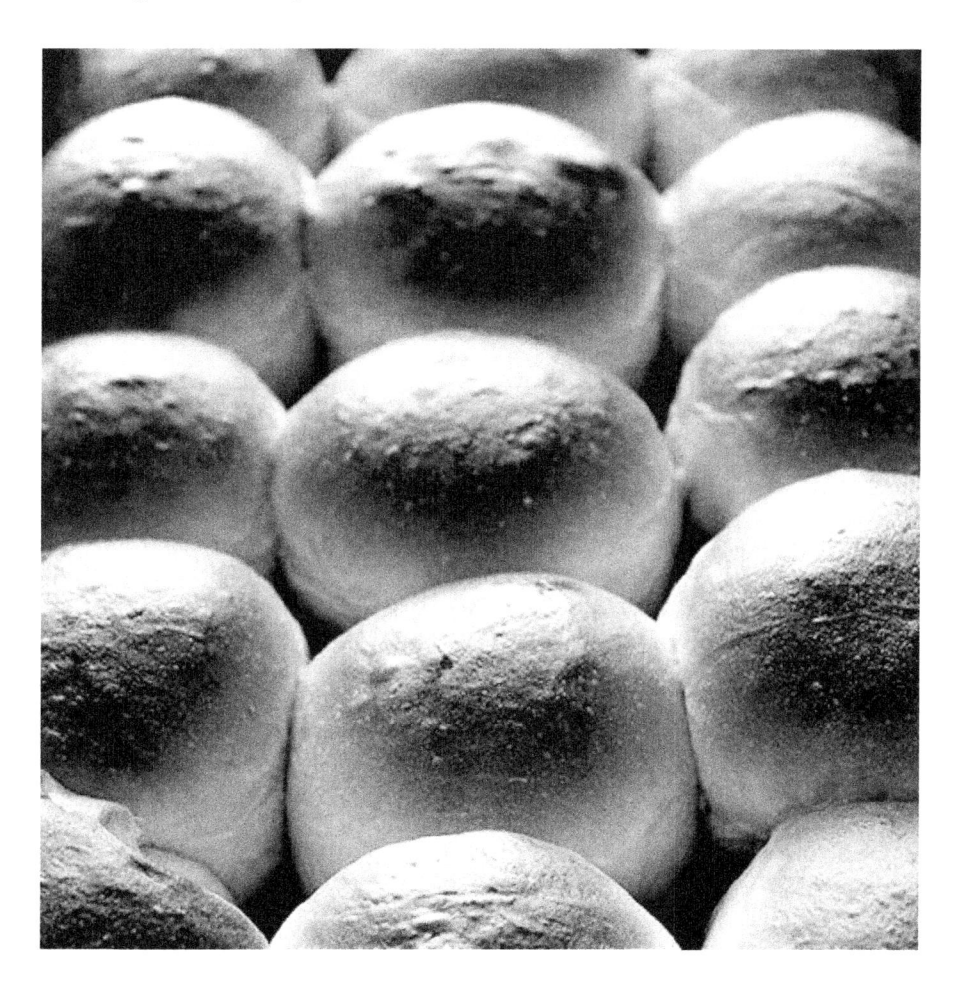

Ingredients
- 300ml (1 ¼ cups) warm milk
- 1 tablespoon honey
- ¾ teaspoon vanilla extract, unsweetened
- 60ml (¼ cup) olive oil
- 1 tablespoon apple cider vinegar
- ½ teaspoon baking powder
- 7g (2 teaspoons) dry active yeast
- 4 tablespoons granulated sugar
- 200g (2 cups) gluten free almond flour / or any other gluten free flour, leveled
- 100g (1 cup) Tapioca / potato starch, leveled
- 2 teaspoons Xanthan Gum
- 1 teaspoon salt
- 3 egg whites, divided
- ¾ teaspoon lemon extract
- ¾ tablespoon molasses

Directions

- According to the manufacturer of your bread machine, into the greased pan of bread machine place all the ingredients, reserve one egg white.
- Select dough / knead / manual cycle to prepare dough and press start.
- When kneading cycle ends, using floured hands transfer dough onto a clean working space,

dusted with flour. Punch down dough, knead for
4-5 times and then divide evenly into 12 pieces.
- Shape each piece into round and place on a 9 by
15 inch greased baking sheets. Cover pan with a
damp towel and let rest in a warm place for 30-
45 minutes or until double in size.
- In the meantime, place baking rack in the top
shelf of oven, set temperature at 350 degrees F
and let preheat.
- In a bowl beat reserve egg white and 1 tablespoon
water until combine and brush over each roll.
- Place baking sheets into oven and bake for 20-25
minutes or until nicely golden brown, switch
sides of pans halfway through baking.
- Cool baked rolls on wire rack completely before
serving.

Nutritional information:

95 Cal, 18 g total fat, 0 mg chol., 85 mg sodium, 15 g
carb., 1 g fiber, 3 g protein.

Calzones

Yield: About 8 rolls
Preparation Time: 1 hour and 10 minutes
Baking Time: 35 minutes

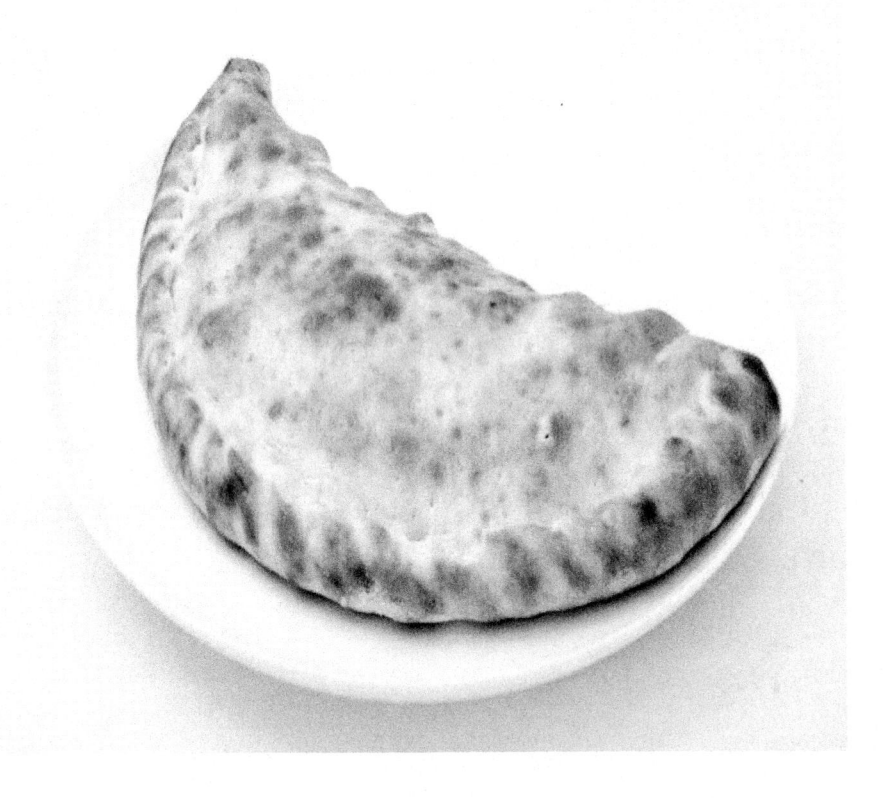

Ingredients
For the bread

- 300ml (1 ¼ cups) warm water

- 60ml (¼ cup) olive oil
- 2 egg whites
- 1 tablespoon apple cider vinegar
- ½ teaspoon baking powder
- 7g (2 teaspoons) dry active yeast
- 2 tablespoons granulated sugar
- 200g (2 cups) gluten free almond flour / or any other gluten free flour, leveled
- 100g (1 cup) Tapioca / potato starch, leveled
- 2 teaspoons Xanthan Gum
- 1 teaspoon salt

For the filling

- 123g (½ cup) pizza sauce
- 57g (½ cup) shredded fat-free mozzarella cheese
- 90g (½ cup) chopped green bell pepper
- 90g (½ cup) sliced pepperoni
- 40g (½ cup) sliced mushrooms

Directions

- According to the manufacturer of your bread machine, into the greased pan of bread machine place all the ingredients, select dough / knead / manual cycle to prepare dough and press start.
- When kneading cycle ends, using floured hands transfer dough onto a clean working space,

dusted with flour. Punch down dough, cover and let rest for 10 minutes.
- In the meantime, place baking rack in the top shelf of oven, set temperature at 400 degrees F and let preheat. Grease a 9 by 15 inch baking sheet and set aside until require.
- Then divide dough evenly into 8 pieces and roll each piece into 6-inch diameter round crust.
- Spread 1 tablespoon of pizza sauce over bottom half of each crust, leave 1 inch edge uncovered.
- Over sauce sprinkle with pepper, pepperoni and mushrooms and fold uncover half over filling to make half circles.
- Seal edges by pinching crust using form and place calzone onto prepared baking sheet.
- Bake calzones for 30-35 minutes until nicely golden brown on all sides.
- Cool baked calzones on cooling rack for 10 minutes before serving.

Nutritional information:

210 Cal, 9 g total fat, 30 mg chol., 450 mg sodium, 22 g carb., 1 g fiber, 11 g protein.

Printed in Great Britain
by Amazon